Contemporary Diagnosis and Management of

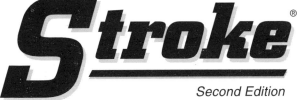

Second Edition

Jesse Weinberger, MD

Professor of Neurology,
Mount Sinai Medical Center,
New York, NY
Chief, Neurology Service,
North General Hospital,
New York, NY

Published by
Handbooks in Health Care Co.,
Newtown, Pennsylvania, USA

International Standard Book Number: 1-884065-85-6

Library of Congress Catalog Card Number: 99-68884

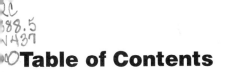

RC
388.5
N437

Table of Contents

This book has been prepared and is presented as a service to the medical community. The information provided reflects the knowledge, experience, and personal opinions of Jesse Weinberger, MD, Professor of Neurology, Mount Sinai Medical Center, New York, NY.

This book is not intended to replace or to be used as a substitute for the complete prescribing information prepared by each manufacturer for each drug. Because of possible variations in drug indications, in dosage information, in newly described toxicities, in drug/drug interactions, and in other items of importance, reference to such complete prescribing information is definitely recommended before any of the drugs discussed are used or prescribed.

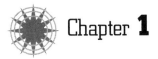 Chapter **1**

Pathophysiology of Cerebrovascular Disease

S troke is an abnormality of brain function caused by disruption of the circulation to the brain lasting more than 24 hours. It is the third leading cause of death in the United States, and is a significant source of disability. The cost is great not only in human suffering, but also in economic terms. Many patients disabled by a stroke consider it a fate worse than death. Therefore, stroke prevention and treatment are critical public health concerns. Recent advances in the understanding of the causes of stroke have made its prevention achievable.

The advent of thrombolytic therapy for acute stroke has changed the outlook from a hopeless condition to a potentially treatable illness, and has raised awareness that stroke should be treated on an emergency basis as a 'brain attack' analogous to the treatment of coronary heart disease. Two different systems must be considered in stroke diagnosis and management: the circulatory system and the nervous system. A disturbance in the circulatory system initiates the damage to brain structures. The location of the brain injury determines the symptoms, signs, and extent of disability of the stroke. Brain structure and chemistry are involved in the susceptibility and propagation of nerve cell damage.

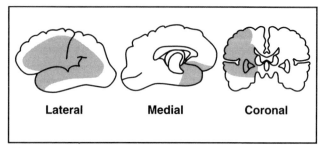

Figure 1: *The distribution of blood circulation to the cerebral hemisphere supplied by the middle cerebral artery to the lateral surface of the brain and basal ganglia. Occlusion of the middle cerebral artery results in contralateral paralysis involving the face and hand more than the leg because of involvement of the inferolateral motor cortex, where these structures are represented.* Figure courtesy of Dr. Paul Anderson.

Circulatory Anatomy

The brain consists of two cerebral hemispheres, with the cerebral cortex surrounding large deep structures: the basal ganglia and thalamus, the white matter tracts ascending and descending from the cortex, and the fluid-filled ventricular system. The cerebral cortex is subdivided into the frontal, parietal, temporal, and occipital lobes. The deep structures of the cerebrum are connected to the brain stem, containing the midbrain, pons, and medulla. The cerebellum lies posterior to the brain stem.

Each cerebral hemisphere is supplied with blood by the internal carotid artery. The right common carotid artery arises from the brachiocephalic trunk, and the left arises from the arch of the aorta. Both common carotid arteries divide in the neck just below the angle of the mandible to form the internal carotid artery to the brain and the external carotid artery to the face. The internal carotid artery courses through the petrous bone and the caver-

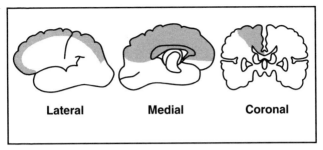

Lateral   **Medial**   **Coronal**

Figure 2: *The distribution of blood circulation to the cerebral hemisphere supplied by the anterior cerebral artery to the medial surface of the brain. Occlusion of the anterior cerebral artery results in contralateral paralysis involving the leg more than the face and hand because of involvement of the superior medial motor cortex, where the leg is represented. Figure courtesy of Dr. Paul Anderson.*

nous sinus toward the eye, where the ophthalmic artery branches off. The anterior choroidal artery branch arises from the internal carotid just before it separates into the middle cerebral and anterior cerebral arteries. The anterior choroidal artery supplies the medial temporal lobe. The middle cerebral artery provides circulation to the lateral surface of the cerebral hemispheres, including the frontal, parietal, and temporal lobes (Figure 1). Small branches from the horizontal portion of the middle cerebral artery—the lenticulostriate arteries—supply the deep structures of the basal ganglia and the internal capsule, which is the white matter of the main connecting pathway between the cortex and lower structures. The anterior cerebral artery provides circulation to the medial surface of the cerebral hemispheres, including the frontal, parietal, and temporal lobes (Figure 2).

The brain stem is supplied by the two vertebral arteries, which arise from the subclavian arteries on each side

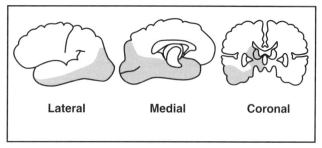

| Lateral | Medial | Coronal |

Figure 3: *The distribution of blood circulation to the cerebral hemisphere supplied by the posterior cerebral artery, the terminal branch of the basilar artery. Occlusion of the posterior cerebral artery results in contralateral loss of vision because of involvement of the occipital lobe, which mediates vision. Figure courtesy of Dr. Paul Anderson.*

and join to form the basilar artery. The posterior inferior cerebellar artery arises from the proximal intracranial vertebral artery to provide circulation to the inferior cerebellum and the lateral medulla. The anterior cerebellar artery and superior cerebellar artery arise from the basilar artery to supply the rest of the brain stem and cerebellum, along with small penetrating arteries from the basilar. The terminal branches of the basilar artery are the posterior cerebral arteries, which supply the occipital lobe and the posterior portions of the parietal and temporal lobes, as well as the thalamus (Figure 3).

An extensive network of collateral anastomoses supplies blood to regions of the brain that may be deprived of their primary blood supply because of occlusion of a major vessel. The main collateral channel is the circle of Willis at the base of the brain (Figure 4). The two carotid arteries communicate from side to side through the anterior communicating artery. Each carotid artery communicates with the posterior cerebral artery through the posterior communicating artery, producing a collateral

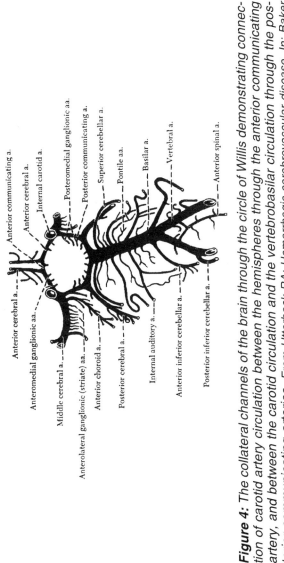

Anterior communicating a.

Anterior cerebral a.

Internal carotid a.

Posteromedial ganglionic aa.

Posterior communicating a.

Superior cerebellar a.

Pontile aa.

Basilar a.

Vertebral a.

Anterior cerebral a.

Anteromedial ganglionic aa.

Middle cerebral a.

Anterolateral ganglionic (striate) aa.

Anterior choroid a.

Posterior cerebral a.

Internal auditory a.

Anterior inferior cerebellar a.

Posterior inferior cerebellar a.

Anterior spinal a.

Figure 4: The collateral channels of the brain through the circle of Willis demonstrating connection of carotid artery circulation between the hemispheres through the anterior communicating artery, and between the carotid circulation and the vertebrobasilar circulation through the posterior communicating arteries. From Utterback RA: Hemorrhagic cerebrovascular disease. In: Baker AB, Baker LH: Clinical Neurology. Harper and Row, 1977, Chapter 11. Used with permission.

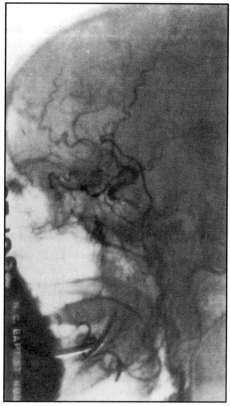

Figure 5: *Collateral flow from the external carotid artery in a patient with a complete occlusion of the internal carotid artery demonstrated by contrast angiography. The cerebral hemisphere is supplied by retrograde flow through the ophthalmic artery into the internal carotid artery and connections between the distal middle cerebral arteries and leptomeningeal vessels from the middle meningeal artery.* From Toole JF: Ischemic cerebrovascular disease. In: Baker AB, Baker LH: Clinical Neurology. Harper & Row, 1977, Chapter 10. Used with permission.

pathway between the cerebral and the vertebrobasilar circulations. Collateral channels can also arise between the external carotid artery and the internal carotid artery when the internal carotid artery is occluded. Blood from the supraorbital branch of the external carotid artery can flow retrograde through the ophthalmic artery to fill the internal carotid artery, and the meningeal branches of the external carotid artery can anastomose with distal branches of the cerebral arteries (Figure 5). Watershed areas of brain circulation occur at the confluences of distal branches of the cerebral arteries, at the junction of the middle and anterior cerebral artery territories in the midportion of the hemispheres, and at the junction of the middle and posterior cerebral arteries in the posterior parietal lobe. These areas are more vulnerable to ischemia with sudden drops in perfusion pressure.

Vascular Etiology of Ischemic Cerebrovascular Disease

The two main categories of cerebrovascular disease are ischemic and hemorrhagic. Ischemic infarction occurs from reduction of blood supply to a brain region because of occlusive disease of the blood vessel supplying that territory. Hemorrhagic vascular disease occurs when a blood vessel to the brain ruptures. About 85% of strokes are ischemic, and 15% are hemorrhagic.[1,2]

Ischemic strokes are subdivided into large-vessel thrombotic strokes, small-vessel thrombotic strokes, atheroembolic strokes from large arteries to distal branches, and cardioembolic strokes.[1,2] Extracranial atherosclerotic vascular disease, primarily at the carotid artery bifurcation, accounts for about 20% of ischemic strokes. Intracranial vascular disease accounts for about 30% of ischemic strokes, and cardioembolic disease accounts for about 20%. Etiology cannot be determined in about 30% of cases, and these are termed cryptogenic strokes (Figures 6 and 7).

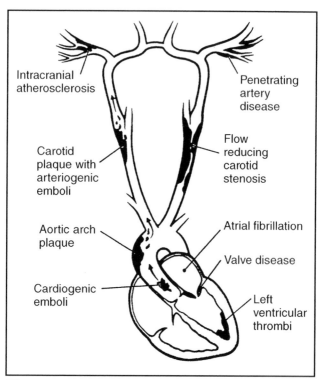

Figure 6: *Anatomy of cerebral ischemic stroke demonstrating cardioembolic sources, atherothrombotic and hemodynamic disease from the carotid bifurcation, intracranial atherosclerosis, and small intracranial vascular disorders.[1] Used with permission.*

Mechanisms of Ischemic Stroke
Intracranial Thrombosis

Ischemic strokes from intracranial vascular disease usually involve the deep structures of the brain in the region of the basal ganglia, thalamus, and internal capsule (Figure 8). Small infarcts called lacunae (holes) are mainly

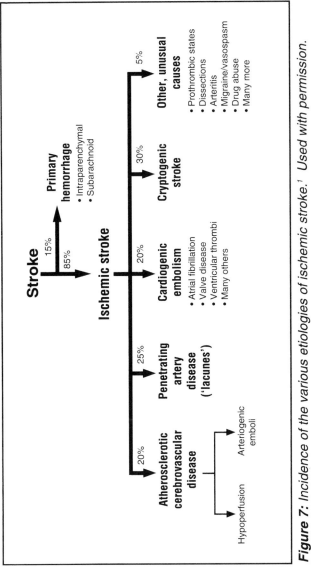

Figure 7: *Incidence of the various etiologies of ischemic stroke.[1] Used with permission.*

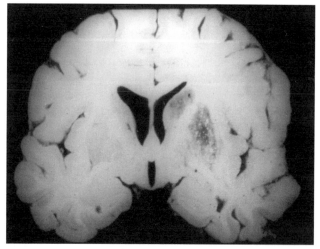

Figure 8: *A cerebral infarction involving the basal ganglia and internal capsule in the deep structures of the cerebral hemisphere. Deep infarctions more commonly result from occlusive vascular disease, and usually produce a bland or white infarction without hemorrhage.* From Weinberger J: Current management strategies for cerebrovascular stenosis: prophylaxis and treatment. In: Peterson PL, Phillis JW: Novel Therapies for CNS Injuries: Rationales and Results. *Boca Raton, Fla, CRC Press, 1996, pp 69-88.*

caused by proliferative changes in the walls of arterioles (lipohyalinization), which lead to fibrinoid necrosis and thrombosis of the vessels[3] (Figure 9). These proliferative changes in arterioles are primarily caused by hypertension and diabetes, which are major risk factors for stroke. A small lacunar infarct in a critical white matter pathway can cause significant neurologic deficit, while the brains of hypertensive patients examined at postmortem may have multiple small lacunar strokes that remained asymptomatic, or perhaps caused mild cognitive changes during

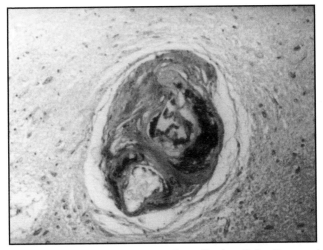

Figure 9: *Fibrinoid necrosis from lipohyalinization and thickening of the wall of a small intracranial artery in the deep structures of the brain, with resultant thrombosis of the lumen. These lesions usually result from hypertension and diabetes, and are associated with small lacunar infarctions in the deep structures of the brain. From Weinberger J, as in Figure 8.*

life. Occlusion of larger intracranial vessels may cause larger strokes. Atherosclerotic disease of the intracranial vessels is more common in African and Asian patients than in Caucasians.[4]

Extracranial Atherosclerosis

Atherosclerotic disease at the carotid artery bifurcations can cause stroke by artery-to-artery embolization, or by acute thrombosis with reduction in distal perfusion (Figure 10). The mechanism of production of atherosclerosis has been studied primarily in the coronary arteries, but is also applicable to the carotid arteries. Phase 1 of the atherosclerotic process involves thickening of the intima.

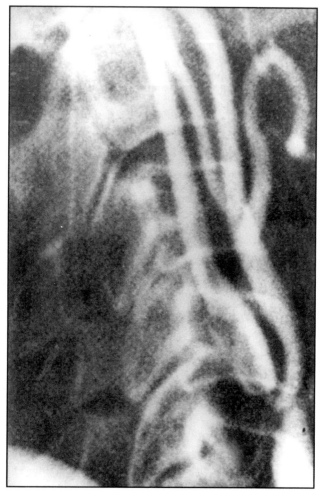

Figure 10: An atherosclerotic plaque at the carotid artery bifurcation causing narrowing of both the carotid sinus and the origin of the internal carotid artery, a major source of embolic cerebral infarction. *From Weinberger J, as in Figure 8.*

The earliest atherosclerotic lesion, type I, is the fatty streak, which is formed by macrophages containing lipid droplets.[5] These lesions arise at points of curvature or branching in arteries because of sheer stresses. The posterior wall of the carotid bifurcation opposite the origin of the external carotid artery is the chief site of atherosclerotic deposition because of turbulent flow with eddy currents and flow reversals causing deposition of lipid material. Type II lesions occur when macrophages and extracellular lipid proliferate in the area of the fatty streak.[6] Type III lesions develop with propagation of smooth-muscle cells stimulated by fibroblast growth factor, platelet growth factor, and angiotensin II.[7]

Phase 2 of the atherosclerotic process involves the formation of exophytic plaque. Lipid can accumulate extracellularly with a confluent cellular component (type IV), or the lipid can be concentrated in a central core with a thin fibrous cap (type Va). These plaques are prone to rupture, causing intraplaque hemorrhage (acute phase 3), which in the coronary arteries can occlude the vessel (acute phase 4), even though the original plaque did not cause a significant stenosis.[5] The coronary arteries can also occlude when collagen is deposited in the plaque after thrombus formation, causing thickening of the wall from fibrosis (type Vb), which can lead to occlusion (phase 5).[5]

The same process appears to occur in the carotid artery bifurcation in the initial phase of intimal thickening.[8] Symptoms of stroke and transient ischemic attack (TIA) associated with carotid artery disease mainly occur with acute plaque rupture and hemorrhage into the plaque, with resultant embolization. These occlude distal intracranial branches or the internal carotid artery.[9-11]

Cardioembolic Stroke

Cardioembolic stroke usually produces infarction in the distal intracranial vessels involving the cerebral cortex.[12] Most middle cerebral artery occlusions are found on patho-

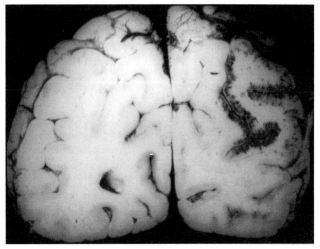

Figure 11: *A hemorrhagic or red infarct in the cerebral cortex. Distal infarction in the cerebral cortex is usually secondary to embolic events, most often from a cardiac source. Hemorrhage of varying degrees into the area of infarction almost always occurs when reperfusion of blood occurs. From Weinberger J, as in Figure 8.*

logic examination to be cardioembolic.[13] Almost all cardioembolic infarctions are associated with some degree of hemorrhagic transformation, which occurs up to 48 hours after the onset of stroke when recanalization or disintegration of the embolic clot occurs, and blood supply is restored to the friable infarcted tissue (Figure 11). The most common cause of cardiogenic embolism is atrial fibrillation. The risk of stroke is increased 17-fold in patients with atrial fibrillation and valvular rheumatic heart disease, compared to matched controls.[14] Nonvalvular atrial fibrillation is much more common, and also increases the risk of stroke 6-fold compared to matched controls, with the highest incidence in people over age 75.[14]

Embolic strokes can also occur in association with acute myocardial infarction,[12] particularly with involvement of the anterior wall.[15] The risk continues from about 48 hours after infarction to about 6 months, after which the damaged myocardial wall becomes akinetic, and is less likely to cause embolization of thrombus.[15] Stroke has been associated with mitral valve prolapse,[16] which occurs in up to 10% of the general population, but has been documented in case-controlled studies to increase the risk of cardioembolic stroke. Patent foramen ovale is a common abnormality in the general population, but has also been documented as the source of paradoxic brain embolism when clots from the peripheral veins pass from the right to the left side of the heart without being filtered by the lung.[17]

Bacterial endocarditis, both acute and subacute, can cause embolic brain infarction in the infection of a rheumatic or prosthetic valve, but subacute bacterial endocarditis can occur in elderly patients with no known valvular heart disease.[18] Noninfected patients with prosthetic mechanical heart valves are at high risk for cardioembolic events, while patients with porcine valve replacements are at lower risk. Cardioembolic stroke has also been associated with mitral annulus calcification and atrial septal aneurysms, but the relative risk of these abnormalities has not been definitively established.

Another cause of stroke classified as cardioembolic is atherosclerotic plaque in the arch of the aorta.[19] These plaques, however, are really a source of atheroembolic brain infarction similar to plaques at the carotid artery bifurcation. Amarenco et al documented a significantly increased frequency of ulcerated atherosclerotic plaques of the aortic arch of stroke patients on postmortem examination,[20] as well as an association with stroke in patients with aortic arch plaques more than 4 mm thick on examination with transesophageal echocardiography.[21]

Coagulation and Stroke

Hematologic abnormalities and coagulopathies are associated with an increased risk of ischemic stroke. Polycythemia increases the risk of stroke, whether from hyperviscosity of the blood, or increased platelet activity causing thrombosis.[22,23] Stroke is associated with deficiencies in the naturally occurring anticoagulant proteins antithrombin III, protein C, and protein S.[24,25] Hyperaggregable platelets lead to intracranial thrombosis in thrombotic thrombocytopenic purpura, which also can result in intracranial hemorrhage when platelets are depleted.[26] Anticardiolipin antibody and the lupus anticoagulant have been identified as significant independent risk factors for stroke, equivalent to hypertension and diabetes, without the presence of other manifestations of collagen vascular disorder.[27] Sickle cell disease is associated with both intracranial and extracranial vasculopathy caused by inspissation of the sickle cells into the arterial wall, resulting in thrombosis.[28] Diabetes is associated with increased platelet aggregability and serum hypercoagulability, which can contribute to stroke.[29]

Hemorrhagic Stroke

The large blood vessels to the brain travel in the subarachnoid space between the pia mater and the arachnoid. The arterioles penetrate the brain parenchyma, though a membranous separation still exists, forming the blood-brain barrier. Intraparenchymal hemorrhage, which results from rupture of intracranial arterioles, accounts for 75% of intracranial hemorrhage, and subarachnoid hemorrhage accounts for 25%. The main cause of intracranial hemorrhage is hypertension, which causes microaneurysms to form on the walls of arterioles damaged by lipohyalinization.[30] Intraparenchymal hemorrhage usually occurs in the deep structures of the brain in the region of the basal ganglia. Lobar hemorrhage can also result from hypertension, but it often is caused by amyloid angiopathy, particularly in the elderly.[31]

Subarachnoid hemorrhage most commonly occurs from rupture of saccular aneurysms that form at branching points of the intracranial arteries at the circle of Willis, frequently involving the origin of the posterior communicating arteries, anterior communicating arteries, and middle cerebral arteries. Arteriovenous malformations, in which cerebral arteries flow directly into veins without passing through a capillary bed, can also cause subarachnoid hemorrhage, although they often present as a mass lesion with progressive focal neurologic deficit and seizure disorder. Venous abnormalities, such as cavernous hemangioma or venous angioma, rarely cause subarachnoid or intraparenchymal hemorrhage.

The Brain in Cerebral Ischemia

Reduction in blood supply to the brain below a critical level results in brain infarction. The normal rate of blood flow to the gray matter, which consists mainly of neuron cell bodies, is 50 to 70 mL/100 g of tissue/minute.[32] In the white matter, which mainly consists of axons (long projections of the nerve cell that communicate with other nerve cells) covered by a fatty sheath called myelin, the flow is 10 to 20 mL/100 g/minute.[32] Cerebral blood flow is maintained at a fairly constant level over a wide range of mean blood pressure, from 60 to 160 mm Hg, by a process called autoregulation, in which brain arterioles dilate and decrease resistance when the mean blood pressure is low, and constrict to increase resistance when the mean pressure is elevated.[33]

At higher and lower pressures, blood flow changes linearly with blood pressure. Cerebral blood flow also responds to changes in partial pressure of carbon dioxide (PCO_2), with a 4% change in cerebral blood flow for each mm Hg change in PCO_2. This ensures that blood flow is increased to regions of demand, so that blood flow is increased to where the brain is actively metabolizing. However, in significant ischemia, autoregulation is lost and blood flow increases or decreases with changes in blood pressure, but does not respond to changes in PCO_2. When blood flow decreases below 20 mL/100 g/minute, neurons cease to function, but are still viable. When blood flow decreases below 10 mL/100 g per minute for 30 minutes, irreversible neuronal damage occurs.[34] When a cerebral artery is occluded, blood flow in the region in the center of the arterial territory is reduced below the critical level, but regions immediately surrounding the center may have insufficient blood flow to maintain neuronal function and still be viable. This region is known as the ischemic penumbra.[35]

The primary source of energy production in the brain is aerobic metabolism of glucose.[36] The brain also stores energy in the form of phosphocreatine (PC), which can temporarily provide energy in hypoxia or ischemia when aerobic metabolism cannot be maintained.[36] The brain is capable of anaerobic metabolism, but this does not provide sufficient adenosine triphosphate (ATP) energy to sustain brain function, and also produces lactate,[37] which causes a regional acidosis that is toxic to neurons.[38] For this reason, hyperglycemia at the onset of cerebral ischemia in animal models produces a greater degree of ischemic damage than does hypoglycemia, because of increased levels of lactate buildup.[39]

When high-energy phosphate stores of ATP and PC in the brain are depleted, the neurons can no longer maintain the membrane potential necessary for retaining potassium within cells, and for preventing sodium influx. This causes an influx of sodium and water into the cells, causing swelling of the neurons, which produces cytotoxic edema of the ischemic brain region.[40] When cells undergo necrosis, proteases and lipases are extruded into the surrounding brain parenchyma, causing destruction of the neuropil, and interstitial vasogenic edema.[40]

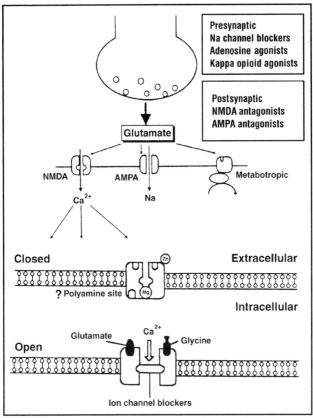

Figure 12: The excitotoxic cascade, leading to cerebral ischemic neuronal death through stimulation of the NMDA and AMPA receptors by the excitatory amino acids glutamate and aspartate.[42]

Energy depletion also causes release of neurotransmitters, the molecules involved in transmission of information from one neuron to another through the synapse (a space connecting the neurons). High concentrations of extracellular neurotransmitters can be toxic to neurons.

The amino acid glutamate is excitatory to neurons and causes excitotoxic damage, leading to neuronal death in ischemia.[41] Stimulation of AMPA receptors initially causes further influx of sodium into neurons, along with increased cellular edema. However, this change does not result in irreversible neuronal death.[42] Irreversible neuronal death is associated with overstimulation of N-methyl-D-aspartate (NMDA) receptors, which causes calcium influx into cells[43] (Figure 12). Intracellular calcium appears to be the final common pathway for ischemic neuronal death, with stimulation of lipases that release free fatty acids that can initiate lipid peroxidation, and of proteases that destroy the proteins of the neuron.[43]

When the striatum becomes ischemic, massive release of dopamine occurs.[44] Depletion of dopamine before the onset of ischemia protects the striatum from neuronal damage,[45,46] and also protects the surrounding white matter.[47]

Nitric oxide (NO) and peroxynitrite, a free radical formed from NO in the presence of superoxide radicals, are also implicated in ischemic neuronal death.[48] In the presence of NO, DNA fragmentation caused by ischemia induces activity of poly(ADP-ribose) polymerase (PARP), a nuclear protein involved in DNA repair.[48,49] PARP activity depletes energy reserves by consuming ADP and NAD to repair the DNA, thus contributing to cell death by energy failure.[48,49] Mice cloned without the gene for PARP are resistant to ischemic neuronal damage.[48,49]

Neuronal death in ischemia is delayed even though the ischemic cascade is immediately set into motion,[36,43] and neurons do not show pathologic signs of necrosis until 8 hours after stroke onset.[50] The neurons can be salvaged from necrosis within 3 hours with NMDA antagonists such as MK 801 or dextrorphan.[51] However, in severe ischemia, even if necrosis is prevented, apoptosis—a programmed cell death dependent on DNA synthesis—can still occur, causing shrinkage and destruction of neurons.[52]

Several regions of the brain are selectively vulnerable to uniform decrements in cerebral blood flow, particularly the CA1 cell layer of the hippocampus, small neurons in the striatum, and cellular layer IV of the cerebral neocortex. These neurons undergo ischemic necrosis even though the neurons around them are preserved.[50] Nerve terminals that secrete neurotransmitters also are selectively vulnerable to ischemia. Dopamine and norepinephrine neurons are more sensitive than serotonin, glutamate, and gamma-aminobutyric acid neurons.[53,54]

In ischemia, the presence of small amounts of blood and oxygen may actually contribute to ischemic damage. Incomplete ischemia with less than 10 mL/100 g/minute produces a greater degree of ischemic damage than when blood is eliminated completely. In a gerbil carotid occlusion model, oxygen is sufficient to maintain metabolism of dopamine to dihydroxyphenylacetic acid by monoamine oxidase for up to 4 hours after onset of ischemia.[55] This reaction requires molecular oxygen and produces hydrogen peroxide, suggesting that oxygen is sufficient to produce neuronal damage from oxidative stress and lipid peroxidation.

Reperfusion of blood into a damaged ischemic area also may contribute to neuronal injury. Because autoregulation is lost in ischemia, reperfusion can result in a syndrome of luxury perfusion, in which hyperemia occurs in areas of infarction.[56] This can lead to increased vasogenic edema, or even hemorrhage into the infarction. White blood cells are also delivered to the infarcted tissue, and can increase the amount of damage to the neuropil by lipid peroxidation of the damaged tissue.[57]

Symptoms of Brain Ischemia

Stroke symptoms usually occur acutely, but sometimes evolve progressively over hours to days. Strokes with maximal acute symptoms that start to resolve most often arise from an embolic source, while strokes that progress over time more often result from thrombosis of an artery.[58] Symptoms occasionally resolve completely within 24 hours, in which case the episode is classified as a TIA. Resolution of symptoms within 48 hours is classified as a reversible ischemic neurologic deficit (RIND). Most TIAs resolve within 1 hour. Those that last longer than 4 hours have a pathophysiology more similar to RINDs.[59]

The symptoms associated with stroke are related to the involved region of the brain. When the middle cerebral artery is occluded, the contralateral face and arm develop more paralysis than the leg because, in the human homunculus, the face and arm are represented on the lateral inferior surface of the brain, while the leg is represented in the midline (Figure 1). Conversely, when the anterior cerebral artery is occluded, the leg is more involved than the arm (Figure 2). Occlusions of the posterior cerebral artery produce occipital lobe infarction with a contralateral hemianopia (visual field defect) (Figure 3). Visual field defects can also occur in posterior temporal lesions with a superior quadrantanopia, or in posterior parietal lesions with an inferior quadrantanopia, from involvement of the optic tract from the optic chiasm to the geniculate bodies, or the optic radiation from the geniculate bodies to the occipital lobe.

Frontal lobe lesions produce contralateral paralysis. Lesions in the parietal lobe produce contralateral sensory loss, particularly sensations requiring cortical function (eg, joint position sense, proprioception [location of the limbs in space], and stereognosis [recognizing objects by touch]). Temporal lobe lesions in the dominant hemisphere, usually the left (even in left-handed individuals), produce aphasia (difficulty with speech).[60] Anterior temporal lesions produce expressive aphasia with inability to speak fluently and difficulty naming objects. Posterior temporal lesions produce receptive aphasia with difficulty understanding the speech of others, but preserved ability to speak fluently, although the speech might not be relevant. Lesions in the dominant hemisphere not directly involving the speech centers in the temporal lobe can still cause difficulty expressing thoughts, even though speech can be produced or phrases repeated (transcortical aphasia). Lesions of the nondominant hemisphere (usually the right), particularly involving the parietal lobe, can produce extinction of the opposite side of the body, in which that side of the body is partially or totally ignored. The patient may even deny having a stroke.[61]

Infarcts in the deep structures of the brain can produce symptoms of paralysis, sensory loss, aphasia, and hemianopia by involvement of the white matter tracts that deliver information to and from the cortical regions of the brain. Lacunar strokes in the white matter tracts typically present with four characteristic syndromes: dysarthria clumsy hand, ataxic hemiparesis, pure motor stroke, and pure sensory stroke.[4]

Brain stem strokes are distinguished by cranial nerve abnormalities on the ipsilateral side of the face, and paralysis on the opposite side of the body because the pyramidal tracts descending from the frontal lobe cross over to innervate the contralateral side of the body at the level of the lower medulla. Typical findings in conjunction with a contralateral hemiparesis are: (1) an ipsilateral oculomotor (third) nerve palsy, with ptosis (droop of the eyelid), dilation of the pupil, and inability to move the eye medially, upward or downward; (2) an abducens (sixth) nerve palsy with inability to move the eye laterally, often associated with a lower motor neuron facial (seventh) nerve palsy in which the eye cannot be closed and the upper lip droops; or (3) ipsilateral conjugate paralysis of movement of both eyes toward the lesion, so the eyes are deviated contralaterally toward the side of the extremity paralysis. The presence of nystagmus (shaking of the eyes with a fast and slow component), particularly in the vertical plane, indicates brain stem dysfunction. Brain stem and cerebellar involvement often produce ataxia of the limbs or truncal ataxia with unsteady gait, and can produce dysarthria (slurred speech with normal content).

Occlusion of a vertebral artery or its main branch, the posterior inferior cerebellar artery, can produce the lateral medullary syndrome, with vertigo and nystagmus, nausea and vomiting, loss of pin prick sensation on the ipsilateral side of the face and contralateral side of the body, and difficulty in swallowing and phonation because of paralysis of the ipsilateral vocal cord. Proximal basilar artery occlusion can be devastating, with resultant quadraparesis in an awake patient or, sometimes, stupor and coma. Involvement of the top of the basilar artery can produce bilateral visual loss because of loss of blood supply in both posterior cerebral arteries to the occipital lobe.

Atypical Causes of Stroke

Although most strokes are caused by atherosclerosis, cardiogenic emboli, and hypertensive vascular disease, abnormalities of the vascular supply to the brain can be caused by inflammation, structural abnormalities, or trauma. Inflammatory changes in the large arteries emanating from the aortic arch—Takayasu's arteritis—can cause occlusions of the common carotid arteries or subclavian arteries that give rise to the vertebral arteries, causing ischemic stroke because of hypoperfusion.[62] Takayasu's arteritis mainly occurs in young women, predominantly Asians. Occlusion of the intracranial internal carotid artery in the region of the carotid siphon or cavernous sinus also can occur in the same population, giving rise to a cloudlike pattern of collateral blood vessels filling the cerebral hemisphere. This condition, moyamoya disease, may also be inflammatory, and can cause ischemic stroke because of the carotid occlusive disease, or hemorrhage because of the abnormal vasculature.[63]

Inflammation of the intracranial vasculature involving medium and small arteries can occur in collagen vascular disorders (eg, lupus erythematosus, polyarteritis nodosa).

In the case of lupus erythematosus, stroke can occur because of hypercoagulability secondary to the lupus anticoagulant, or can result from the vasculitis. However, in lupus vasculitis, no distinct occlusive abnormalities are seen on pathologic examination of the brain, yet brain blood flow can be reduced by the inflammatory process.[64] In lupus erythematosus, venous sinus thrombosis or cortical vein thrombosis can occur, causing ischemia because of inability to clear the capillary bed and resultant obstruction of arterial flow.[65] Venous thrombosis is also associated with pregnancy, particularly postpartum. An intrinsic granulomatous angiitis of the central nervous system also can occur, producing ischemic infarction as well as headache.[66] Hemorrhage occasionally occurs from rupture of inflamed vessels. Vasculitis or vasculopathy of intracranial vessels also is associated with intravenous use of cocaine or amphetamine.[67] Spasm of arteries also can occur, particularly in patients with migraine, and can cause cerebral ischemia and infarction.[68]

Dissection of the media of the carotid or vertebral arteries also can lead to vascular occlusion and stroke. Dissection can be attributable to trauma or to congenital medial cystic necrosis of the artery wall.[69] When the wall of the media tears away, hemorrhage between the layers of the media develops in a false lumen that can expand and compromise the flow of blood in the true lumen of the artery, resulting in brain ischemia.

Conclusion

Ischemic stroke can be caused by thrombosis or embolic occlusion of extracranial and intracranial arteries. A critical reduction of blood supply to the brain initiates an ischemic cascade of biochemical events, which leads to the ultimate necrosis of neurons, but can be at least partly reversed within 3 hours. Brain ischemia can be temporary and result in a TIA. The symptoms and signs associated with the stroke are related to the affected region of the brain. Hemorrhage can occur into the brain parenchyma, mainly from hypertension, or into the subarachnoid space from saccular aneurysms and arteriovenous malformation.

References

1. Sherman DG, Dyken ML Jr, Gent M, et al: Antithrombotic therapy for cerebrovascular disorders. An update. *Chest* 1995; 108:444S-456S.

2. Bogousslavsky J, Van Melle G, Regli F: The Lausanne Stroke Registry: analysis of 1,000 consecutive patients with first stroke. *Stroke* 1988;19:1083-1092.

3. Fisher CM: Lacunes: small deep cerebral infarcts. *Neurology* 1965;15:774-778.

4. Caplan LR, Gorelick PB, Hier DB: Race, sex and occlusive cerebrovascular disease: a review. *Stroke* 1986;17:648-655.

5. Fuster V: Coronary artery disease: a clinical-pathological correlation. In: Fuster V, ed. *Syndromes of Atherosclerosis. Correlations of Clinical Imaging and Pathology.* Armonk, NY, Futura, 1996, pp 1-15.

6. Zarins CK, Giddens DP, Bharadvaj BK, et al: Carotid bifurcation atherosclerosis. Quantitative correlation of plaque localization with flow velocity profiles and wall shear stress. *Circ Res* 1983;53:502-514.

7. O'Brien ER, Schwartz SM: A new view of restenosis. In: Fuster V, ed. *Syndromes of Atherosclerosis. Correlation of Clinical Imaging and Pathology.* Armonk, NY, Futura, 1996, pp 485-505.

8. Bond MG, Barnes RW, Riley WA, et al: High-resolution B-mode ultrasound scanning methods in the Atherosclerosis Risk in Communities (ARIC) cohort. *J Neuroimaging* 1991;1:168-172.

9. Imparato AM, Riles TS, Gorstein F: The carotid bifurcation plaque: pathologic findings associated with cerebral ischemia. *Stroke* 1979;10:238-245.

10. Imparato AM, Riles TS, Mintzer R, et al: The importance of hemorrhage in the relationship between gross morphologic characteristics and cerebral symptoms in 376 carotid artery plaques. *Ann Surg* 1983;197:195-203.

11. Lusby RJ, Ferrell LD, Ehrenfeld WK, et al: Carotid plaque hemorrhage. Its role in production of cerebral ischemia. *Arch Surg* 1982;117:1479-1488.

12. Easton JD, Sherman DG: Management of cerebral embolism of cardiac origin. *Stroke* 1980;11:433-442.

13. Lhermitte F, Gautier JC, Derouesne C: Nature of occlusions of the middle cerebral artery. *Neurology* 1970;20:82-88.

14. Wolf PA, Dawber TR, Thomas HE Jr, et al: Epidemiologic assessment of chronic atrial fibrillation and risk of stroke: the Framingham Study. *Neurology* 1978;28:973-977.

15. Asinger RW: Incidence of left-ventricular thrombosis after acute transmural myocardial infarction. Serial evaluation by two-dimensional echocardiography. *N Engl J Med* 1981;305:297-302.

16. Barnett HJ, Boughner DR, Taylor DW, et al: Further evidence relating mitral-valve prolapse to cerebral ischemic events. *N Engl J Med* 1980;302:139-144.

17. Jeanrenaud X, Kappenberger L: Patent foramen ovale and stroke of unknown origin. *Cerebrovasc Dis* 1991;1:184-192.

18. Kanter MC, Hart RG: Neurologic complications of infective endocarditis. *Neurology* 1991;41:1015-1020.

19. Tunick PA, Kronzon I: Protruding atherosclerotic plaque in the aortic arch of patients with systemic embolization: a new finding seen by transesophageal echocardiography. *Am Heart J* 1990;120:658-660.

20. Amarenco P, Duyckaerts C, Tzourio C, et al: The prevalence of ulcerated plaques in the aortic arch in patients with stroke. *N Engl J Med* 1992;326:221-225.

21. Amarenco P, Cohen A, Tzourio C, et al: Atherosclerotic disease of the aortic arch and the risk of ischemic stroke. *N Engl J Med* 1994;331:1474-1479.

22. Toghi H, Yamanouchi H, Murakami M, et al: Importance of the hematocrit as a risk factor in cerebral infarction. *Stroke* 1978;9: 369-374.

23. Kannel WB, Gordon T, Wolf PA, et al: Hemoglobin and the risk of cerebral infarction: the Framingham Study. *Stroke* 1972; 3:409-420.

24. Kohler J, Kasper J, Witt I, et al: Ischemic stroke due to protein C deficiency. *Stroke* 1990;21:1077-1080.

25.   D'Angelo A, Vigano-D'Angelo S, Esmon CT, et al: Acquired deficiencies of protein S. Protein S activity during oral anticoagulation, in liver disease, and in disseminated intravascular coagulation. *J Clin Invest* 1988;81:1445-1454.

26.   Silverstein A: Thrombotic thrombocytopenic purpura. The initial neurologic manifestations. *Arch Neurol* 1968;18:358-362.

27.   The Antiphospholipid Antibodies in Stroke Study (APASS) Group: Anticardiolipin antibodies are an independent risk factor for first ischemic stroke. *Neurology* 1993;43:2069-2073.

28.   Russell MO, Goldberg HI, Hodson A, et al: Effect of transfusion therapy on arteriographic abnormalities and on recurrence of stroke in sickle cell disease. *Blood* 1984;63:162-169.

29.   Mayne EE, Bridges JM, Weaver JA: Platelet adhesiveness, plasma fibrinogen and factor 8 levels in diabetes mellitus. *Diabetologia* 1970;6:436-440.

30.   Cole FM, Yates PO: The occurrence and significance of intracerebral micro-aneurysms. *J Pathol Bacteriol* 1967;93:393-411.

31.   Vinters HV: Cerebral amyloid angiopathy. A critical review. *Stroke* 1987;18:311-324.

32.   Obrist WD, Thompson HK Jr, Wang HS, et al: Regional cerebral blood flow estimated by 133-xenon inhalation. *Stroke* 1975;6:245-256.

33.   Strandgaard S, Oleson J, Skinhoj E, et al: Autoregulation of brain circulation in severe arterial hypertension. *Br Med J* 1973; 1:507-510.

34.   Salford LG, Plum F, Brierley JB: Graded hypoxia-oligemia in rat brain. II. Neuropathological alterations and their implications. *Arch Neurol* 1973;29:234-238.

35.   Astrup J, Siesjo BK, Symon L: Thresholds in cerebral ischemia—the ischemic penumbra. *Stroke* 1981;12:723-725.

36.   Siesjo BK: Pathophysiology and treatment of focal cerebral ischemia. Part I: Pathophysiology. *J Neurosurg* 1992;77:169-184.

37.   Salford LG, Plum F, Siesjo BK: Graded hypoxia-oligemia in rat brain. I. Biochemical alterations and their implications. *Arch Neurol* 1973;29:227-233.

38.   Ginsberg MD, Welsh FA, Budd WW: Deleterious effect of glucose pretreatment on recovery from diffuse cerebral ischemia in the cat. I. Local cerebral blood flow and glucose utilization. *Stroke* 1980;11:347-354.

39. Welsh FA, Ginsberg MD, Rieder W, et al: Deleterious effect of glucose pretreatment on recovery from diffuse cerebral ischemia in the cat. II. Regional metabolite levels. *Stroke* 1980;11:355-363.

40. Fishman RA: Brain edema. *N Engl J Med* 1975;293:706-711.

41. Rothman S: Synaptic release of excitatory amino acid neurotransmitter mediates anoxic neuronal death. *J Neurosci* 1984; 4:1884-1891.

42. Muir KW, Lees KR: Clinical experience with excitatory amino acid antagonist drugs. *Stroke* 1995;26:503-513.

43. Siesjo BK: Pathophysiology and treatment of focal cerebral ischemia. Part II: Mechanisms of damage and treatment. *J Neurosurg* 1992;77:337-354.

44. Slivka A, Brannan TS, Weinberger J, et al: Increase in extracellular dopamine in the striatum during cerebral ischemia: a study utilizing cerebral microdialysis. *J Neurochem* 1988; 50:1714-1718.

45. Globus MY, Ginsberg MD, Dietrich WD, et al: Substantia nigra lesion protects against ischemic damage in the striatum. *Neurosci Lett* 1987;80:251-256.

46. Weinberger J, Nieves-Rosa J, Cohen G: Nerve terminal damage in cerebral ischemia: protective effect of alpha-methyl-para-tyrosine. *Stroke* 1985;16:864-870.

47. Weinberger J, Nieves-Rosa J: Monoamine neurotransmitters in the evolution of infarction in ischemic striatum: morphologic correlation. *J Neural Transm* 1988;71:133-142.

48. Eliasson MJ, Sampei K, Mandir AS, et al: Poly(ADP-ribose) polymerase gene disruption renders mice resistant to cerebral ischemia. *Nat Med* 1997;3(10):1089-1095.

49. Enders M, Wang ZQ, Namura S, et al: Ischemic brain injury is mediated by the activation of poly(ADP-ribose) polymerase. *J Cereb Blood Flow Metab* 1997;17:1143-1151.

50. Brown AW, Brierley JB: The earliest alterations in rat neurones and astrocytes after anoxia-ischaemia. *Acta Neuropathol (Berl)* 1973;23:9-22.

51. Park CK, Nehls DG, Graham DI, et al: The glutamate antagonist MK-801 reduces focal ischemic brain damage in the rat. *Ann Neurol* 1988;24:543-551.

52. Linnik MD, Miller JA, Sprinkle-Cavallo J, et al: Apoptotic DNA fragmentation in the rat cerebral cortex induced by perma-

nent middle cerebral artery occlusion. *Brain Res Mol Brain Res* 1995;32:116-124.

53. Weinberger J, Cohen G: The differential effect of ischemia on the active uptake of dopamine, gamma-aminobutyric acid, and glutamate by brain synaptosomes. *J Neurochem* 1982;38:963-968.

54. Weinberger J, Cohen G, Nieves-Rosa J: Nerve terminal damage in cerebral ischemia: greater susceptibility of catecholamine nerve terminals relative to serotonin nerve terminals. *Stroke* 1983; 14:986-989.

55. Weinberger J, Nieves-Rosa J: Metabolism of monoamine neurotransmitters in the evolution of infarction in ischemic striatum. *J Neural Transm* 1987;69:265-275.

56. Lassen NA: The luxury-perfusion syndrome and its possible relation to acute metabolic acidosis localised within the brain. *Lancet* 1966;2:1113-1115.

57. Kochanek PM, Hallenbeck JM: Polymorphonuclear leukocytes and monocytes/macrophages in the pathogenesis of cerebral ischemia and stroke. *Stroke* 1992;23:1367-1379.

58. Mohr JP, Caplan LR, Melski JW, et al: The Harvard Cooperative Stroke Registry: a prospective registry. *Neurology* 1978;28:754-762.

59. Pessin MS, Duncan GW, Mohr JP, et al: Clinical and angiographic features of carotid transient ischemic attacks. *N Engl J Med* 1977;296:358-362.

60. Naeser MA, Hayward RW: Lesion localization in aphasia with cranial computed tomography and the Boston Diagnostic Aphasia Exam. *Neurology* 1978;28:545-551.

61. Kinsbourne M: Mechanisms of neglect: implications for rehabilitation. *Neuropsychol Rehabil* 1994;4:151-153.

62. Hall S, Barr W, Lie JT, et al: Takayasu arteritis. A study of 32 North American patients. *Medicine* 1985;64:89-99.

63. Suzuki J, Takaku A: Cerebrovascular "moyamoya" disease. Disease showing abnormal net-like vessels in base of brain. *Arch Neurol* 1969;20:288-299.

64. Weinberger J, Gordon J, Hodson AK, et al: Effect of intracerebral vasculitis on regional cerebral blood flow. *Arch Neurol* 1979; 36:681-685.

65. Estanol B, Rodriguez A, Conte G, et al: Intracranial venous thrombosis in young women. *Stroke* 1979;10:680-684.

66. Cupps TR, Moore PM, Fauci AS: Isolated angiitis of the central nervous system. Prospective diagnostic and therapeutic experience. *Am J Med* 1983;74:97-105.

67. Caplan LR, Hier DB, Banks G: Current concepts of cerebrovascular disease—stroke: stroke and drug abuse. *Stroke* 1982; 13:869-872.

68. Rothrock JF, Walicke P, Swenson MR, et al: Migrainous stroke. *Arch Neurol* 1988;45:63-67.

69. Hart RG, Easton JD: Dissections of cervical and cerebral arteries. *Neurol Clin* 1983;1:155-182.

Chapter 2

The Diagnosis of Stroke

The initial evaluation of patients with stroke is critical to identify the type of stroke and the patient's clinical status. Stroke must be differentiated from other conditions (eg, brain tumors, subdural hematoma) that can cause symptoms and signs of brain dysfunction similar to stroke. The clinical neurologic examination is most important in determining the extent of the stroke, and often can establish the nature of the stroke. The blood is examined to determine coagulation abnormalities that could contribute to stroke. Imaging of the brain is performed with computed tomography (CT) or magnetic resonance imaging (MRI) to identify the location and size of the stroke, and whether it is ischemic or hemorrhagic. Flow in the arteries supplying the brain can be assessed with carotid duplex and transcranial Doppler ultrasound, and the vessels can be imaged with magnetic resonance angiography (MRA) or spiral CT angiography. The heart is evaluated with electrocardiography (EKG) and echocardiography for potential sources of embolism. Perfusion in the brain is measured by single photon emission computed tomography (SPECT), and metabolism is measured with positron emission tomography (PET) or MRI spectroscopy. The electric activity of the brain is assessed with electroencephalography to identify seizure activity and to help establish level of consciousness in unresponsive patients. Once the necessary information is obtained, appropriate management and treatment can be initiated to potentially improve the patient's condition and prevent subsequent strokes.

Clinical Evaluation of the Stroke Patient

Examination of the Patient

The first step in evaluating stroke patients is to obtain the history of the event. The clinician should ascertain initial symptoms, time and duration of onset, and the presence of progression or improvement. When a patient is unresponsive or cannot speak because of aphasia, a family member or other observer must be questioned. The examiner can establish, from the history, the presence of weakness on one side of the body, difficulty with speech, change in level of consciousness, visual disturbance on one side of the visual field or in one eye, double vision or movement of vision, change in sensation, loss of balance, incoordination of extremities, headache, or dizziness.

Next, a medical history should be obtained to identify factors that could precipitate stroke. Risk factors, including hypertension, diabetes, coronary artery disease, cardiac arrhythmia, cardiac valve dysfunction, hyperlipidemia, and coagulopathy, are identified. A family history of these conditions also helps establish the etiology of the stroke. The review of systems determines the presence of chest pain, shortness of breath, gastrointestinal disorder, or urinary incontinence associated with the stroke.

The general physical examination is performed before the neurologic examination. First, level of consciousness, heartbeat, and airway patency are established to be certain no emergent life support is necessary. Temperature is important because fever may be associated with embolism from endocarditis. Blood pressure should be taken, both to determine whether hypertension is an etiologic factor, and for management of blood pressure during the treatment of stroke. Pulse rate should be examined to determine if it is rapid or irregular, suggesting a possible cardiac arrhythmia such as atrial fibrillation that could be responsible for an embolic event.

Pulse should be palpated at several different sites. Radial pulses are felt to identify any unilateral loss of the pulse, which may indicate a subclavian artery stenosis. This can be associated with subclavian steal syndrome, in which the subclavian artery distal to the vertebral artery is fed by retrograde flow down the vertebral artery from the brain. Cervical carotid artery pulses are examined to identify carotid artery occlusive disease. Superficial temporal and supraorbital pulses are examined because large pulsatile superficial temporal arteries may be present in carotid occlusive disease to supply flow from the external carotid circulation retrograde through the ophthalmic artery to the internal carotid circulation. The femoral, popliteal, dorsum pedis, and posterior tibial pulses also should be identified. Loss of peripheral pulses could indicate multiple embolic events, possibly resulting from systemic cardiogenic embolization that may have caused the stroke.

The heart should be auscultated with the stethoscope to identify murmurs indicating valvular dysfunction, such as mitral stenosis or mitral valve prolapse, that can lead to embolic stroke. The stethoscope is placed at the angle of the jaw to listen for vascular bruits from the carotid artery that can signify occlusive carotid artery disease. The chest should be auscultated to rule out respiratory compromise that can contribute to stroke from hypoxia. The clinician should examine the abdomen to identify any acute obstruction or an abdominal aortic aneurysm. The rectum should be examined, and a stool guaiac performed, to rule out gastrointestinal bleeding that may precipitate a stroke from hypotension. The skin should be examined to identify petechiae or purpura that may indicate a clotting disorder, or platelet dysfunction that may lead to either hemorrhagic or thrombotic stroke.

The neurologic examination begins with evaluation of mental status. Patients are asked to identify their name, the location, the time, and the circumstances. A patient with a nondominant hemisphere stroke may be able to answer questions normally, but may not be aware of the occurrence of a stroke or the presence of weakness of the contralateral (usually left) side of the body. Speech function should be assessed by listening to the patient speak to determine whether speech is fluent. Speech content can be characterized by whether normal words are used, or if inappropriate words that are similar to the word intended but incorrect are used (paraphasia). The patient should be asked to name objects and body parts, and to repeat sentences and follow commands. This establishes the presence of an expressive or receptive aphasia, indicating a dominant hemisphere lesion, usually the left. Recent and long-term memory should be tested by asking about current and past events, and recall tested by asking the patient to remember a series of words or phrases and repeat them 5 minutes later.

Cognitive ability should be assessed by asking the patient to spell a 4- or 5-letter word forward and backward and to perform simple addition and subtraction. Perception can be tested by assessing whether the patient can identify where he or she is touched when more than one part of the body is stimulated. Visuospatial and constructive ability can be examined by asking the patient to draw or copy objects or patterns, or perform functional tasks such as drawing a clock and indicating the time, or demonstrating how to use an appliance such as a toothbrush.

Next, the cranial nerves, pupillary reflexes, extraocular motions, visual fields, and ocular fundi should be examined. In the fundus, flame-shaped hemorrhages in the choroid can occur with subarachnoid or intracranial hemorrhage. Acute increased intracranial pressure can sometimes produce papilledema and retinal hemorrhage. Ipsilateral ischemic changes occur in internal carotid artery occlusion. Eye movements should be observed for nystagmus. Double simultaneous stimulation of the left and right visual fields should be performed to identify subtle visual field deficits.

The motions of the face, tongue, jaw, and palate must be observed. A droop of the mouth alone indicates an upper motor neuron lesion, while a droop of the mouth associated with inability to close the eye or raise the brow indicates a lower motor neuron lesion of the facial nerve or nucleus. An isolated peripheral facial nerve lesion from an inflammatory cause often is mistaken for stroke, but a central nervous system lesion can also produce lower motor neuron facial weakness with other associated neurologic findings, such as contralateral hemiparesis. The patient should be tested for corneal reflex and sensation to pin prick on the face.

Motor examination proceeds by assessing strength and mobility of the muscle groups responsible for the movement of each joint, at the shoulder, elbow, wrist, fingers, hips, knees, ankles, and toes, in flexion and extension. Muscle tone should be tested for flaccidity or rigidity. The sensory modalities of pin prick and temperature, vibration, joint position sense, and stereognosis should be evaluated.

Deep-tendon reflexes at the biceps, triceps, brachioradialis, knees, and ankles should be elicited by tapping the tendon with a reflex hammer. The response to noxious plantar stimulation of the foot should be examined for a positive Babinski's reflex (an abnormal upgoing big toe with fanning of the other toes, instead of a downgoing big toe). Increased reflexes or an upgoing big toe indicate an upper motor neuron lesion, while hyporeflexia indicates a lower motor neuron lesion. However, in patients with peripheral neuropathy with reduced reflexes (eg, in diabetes), hyperreflexia may not develop after an upper motor neuron lesion.

The cerebellar system is examined by asking patients to touch their nose and the examiner's finger repetitively, and asking the patient to move the heel of the foot up and down the opposite shin from the knee to the foot. Gait should be tested if the patient can walk. Swinging of a leg from the hip with the knee rigid indicates spasticity. A broad-based gait, or loss of balance backward or from side to side, indicates cerebellar dysfunction.

The neurologic history and examination should be synthesized to formulate the anatomic localization (Table 1) and possible etiologies of the stroke. Difficulty expressing speech and a right hemiparesis indicate a left cerebral lesion, usually involving the frontal or temporal lobes. A left hemiparesis with extinction of awareness of the left side indicates a right cerebral lesion, often involving the parietal lobe. A homonymous hemianopia indicates that the lesion is posterior to the optic chiasm on the contralateral side of the brain. Difficulty with coordination and cortical sensations of the hand, such as proprioception, joint position sense, stereognosis, or graphesthesia, indicates dysfunction of the contralateral parietal lobe. A crossed syndrome usually occurs in stroke involving the brain stem, with cranial nerve deficits ipsilateral to the lesion, such as lower motor neuron facial weakness (7th nerve) and weakness of abduction of the eye (8th nerve), and a contralateral hemiparesis of the extremities.

Eye movements are critical in determining whether a stroke involves the cerebral hemisphere or the brain stem. In a cerebral lesion affecting conjugate gaze, the eyes cannot be directed to the contralateral side. This results in deviation of the eyes to the left and right hemiparesis with a left cerebral lesion, and deviation of the eyes to the right and left hemiparesis with a right cerebral lesion. In a brain stem lesion involving conjugate horizontal gaze, the eyes cannot be directed to the ipsilateral side. This results in deviation of the eyes to the right and a right hemiparesis for left brain stem lesions, and deviation of the eyes to the left and a left hemiparesis for right brain stem lesions.

The vascular territory of a stroke often can be determined by clinical examination. A patient with a paraly-

Table 1: The NIH Stroke Scale

The neurologic examination is scored with the NIH Stroke Scale to quantify the degree of neurologic dysfunction from the stroke. A high score correlates with a large infarction, even if this is not shown on initial acute imaging study. This scale is used in most clinical trials, and also is critical in assessing patients for acute thrombolytic therapy or anticoagulation. It should be performed in the initial evaluation of all stroke patients. Subsequent examinations help quantify the progress of the patient.

Level of Consciousness

0 = Alert, keenly responsive

1 = Drowsy, arousable by minor stimulation to obey, answer, or respond

2 = Responds only with reflex motor or autonomic effects, or totally unresponsive

Level of Consciousness Question: Patients are asked the month and their age.

0 = Both correct

1 = One correct

2 = Both incorrect, or unable to respond

Level of Consciousness Command: The patient is asked to close the eye and the hand.

0 = Both correct

1 = One correct

2 = Both incorrect, or unable to respond

Best Language: Standard pictures are named.

0 = Normal

1 = Mild to moderate naming errors, word-finding errors, or paraphasias. Impairment of communication by either comprehension or expression.

2 = Severe: fully developed Broca's (expressive) or Wernicke's (receptive) aphasia

3 = Mute or global aphasia

Best Visual: Test vision in each field to finger movement simultaneously.

0 = Normal

1 = Asymmetry

2 = Complete hemianopia

Best Gaze

0 = Full range of eye movements

1 = Partial gaze palsy

2 = Forced deviation or total gaze paresis not overcome by Doll's eye maneuver

Dysarthria

0 = Normal

1 = Mild to moderate slurring of words, can be understood

2 = Speech slurred, unintelligible

(continued on next page)

Table 1: The NIH Stroke Scale *(continued)*

Best Motor Arm: The patient holds the arm out-stretched at 90 degrees.

0 = Limb holds 90 degrees for full 10 seconds

1 = Limb holds 90-degree position, but drifts before full 10 seconds

2 = Limb cannot hold 90-degree position for full 10 seconds, some effort against gravity

3 = Limb falls, no effort against gravity

4 = No movement

Best Motor Leg: The patient elevates the leg at 30 degrees for 5 seconds.

0 = Leg holds 30-degree position for 5 seconds

1 = Leg falls to intermediate position by end of 5 seconds

2 = Leg falls to bed by 5 seconds, some effort against gravity

3 = Leg falls to bed immediately, no resistance against gravity

4 = No movement

sis more involving the face and arm, rather than the leg, usually has a lesion in the middle cerebral artery territory, while a patient with weakness involving the leg more than the arm usually has a lesion in the anterior cerebral artery territory. A patient with a contralateral hemianopia alone or in association with difficulties in cortical sensations, such as proprioception, usually has a stroke involving the posterior cerebral artery territory, the terminating branch of the basilar artery. A patient with vertigo and nystagmus, difficulty swallowing,

Limb Ataxia: Finger-to-nose and heel-to-shin test.

   0 = Absent (no movement of limb)

   1 = Ataxia present in one limb

   2 = Ataxia present in two limbs

Sensory: Pin prick. If level of consciousness is impaired, score only if a grimace or asymmetric withdrawal is present.

   0 = Normal

   1 = Mild to moderate. Patient feels pin prick less sharp, but is aware of being touched

   2 = Severe to total sensation loss, not aware of being touched

Neglect

   0 = No neglect

   1 = Visual, tactile, or auditory hemi-inattention

   2 = Profound hemi-inattention to more than one modality

hoarseness, ipsilateral Horner's syndrome, decreased pinprick sensation on the ipsilateral side of the face and opposite side of the body, and, sometimes, ipsilateral ataxia, usually has a lesion in the ipsilateral vertebral artery or posterior inferior cerebellar artery territory.

The etiology of the stroke often can be determined by the history and physical examination.[1,2] A patient who has sudden severe headache and rapid reduction in level of consciousness with a hemiparesis has probably had an intracerebral hemorrhage. Severe headache with stiff neck

Table 2: The Glasgow Coma Scale

The Glasgow Coma Scale was designed to establish the severity of traumatic brain injury, but can be applied to patients with stroke when level of consciousness is altered. Abnormal flexion responses refer to decorticate rigidity, and extension responses refer to decerebrate rigidity.

Eye opening

Spontaneously	4
To verbal commands	3
To pain	2
No response	1

Best motor response

To verbal command	6
Localizes pain	5
Flexion—withdrawal	4
Flexion—abnormal	3
Extension	2
No response	1

Best verbal response

Oriented and converses	5
Disoriented and converses	4
Inappropriate words	3
Incomprehensible words	2
No response	1

and alteration of level of consciousness, without focal neurologic deficit or with oculomotor nerve paralysis, suggests a subarachnoid hemorrhage. A patient who has acute onset of a right hemiparesis involving the face and arm more than the leg, with head and eyes deviated away from the hemiparesis, and who is lethargic, probably has had a large middle cerebral artery infarct, which is usually cardioembolic,[3] although it can be attributable to carotid occlusive disease. Palpation of an irregularly irregular pulse and absence of some peripheral pulses can establish that the stroke is most likely cardioembolic from atrial fibrillation, while auscultation of a carotid artery bruit can establish that the most likely source is carotid occlusive disease. A severe hemiparesis in a patient who is wide awake and normally responsive suggests a small, lacunar infarct from intracranial small vessel thrombosis in the subcortical white matter, particularly when the patient is hypertensive or diabetic. The finding of one of the typical 'lacunar syndromes'—pure motor hemiparesis, pure sensory stroke, dysarthria, clumsy hand syndrome, or ataxic hemiparesis—also suggests occlusive disease of small intracranial vessels.[4]

Establishing the etiology and severity of the stroke are critical in deciding the appropriate therapy and management of stroke patients. Quantifying the severity of the stroke and degree of brain damage by employing the NIH Stroke Scale (Table 1),[5] the Glasgow Coma Scale (Table 2),[6] and an estimation of the patient's functional disability with ratings such as the Barthel index (Table 3),[7] is valuable for both prognostic and therapeutic purposes. Most clinical trials of therapeutic agents for stroke employ these scales, and indications for treatment are partly based on these scales, particularly when deciding whether to initiate thrombolytic therapy.[8] Therefore, applying these rating scales is becoming increasingly important as part of the initial evaluation of stroke patients.

Laboratory Investigation of Stroke Patients

Basic hematologic and serum chemistry tests are necessary for appropriate management of stroke patients. The complete blood count can identify the presence of an anemia that may contribute to hypoxemia of the cerebral tissue or be an etiologic factor in stroke (eg, sickle cell ane-

Table 3: The Barthel Index

The Barthel index measures functional capacity. Most clinical trials use the Barthel index to measure outcome in terms of the functional lifestyle patients can maintain. The index is also used in evaluation for rehabilitation.

Feeding (0-2 points)

2: Independent

1: Some help necessary (eg, after food is cut)

0: Unable to independently feed/NPO/ nasogastric tube

Moving from wheelchair to bed and returning (0-3 points)

3: Independent in transfer, or does not require wheelchair

2: Needs help, requires supervision

1: Needs great deal of help to get out of chair or bed

0: Bedridden, bedrest

Personal care (0-1 point)

1: Can wash face and hands, comb hair, clean teeth, shave

0: Unable to perform

Getting on and off toilet (0-2 points)

2: Patient can do it and redress

1: Patient needs assistance

0: Unable to perform/catheter/bedpan

Bathing (0-1 point)

1: Patient can use shower, bathtub, or complete sponge bath

0: Needs assistance in bathing

Walking on level surface (0-3 points)

   3: Can walk 50 yards without help.
       Can use cane or brace.

   2: Needs help or supervision of another person to
       walk 50 yards

   1: Unable to walk, able to propel wheelchair

   0: Unable to walk or propel wheelchair

Ascending and descending stairs (0-2 points)

   2: Can go up and down stairs without help
       or supervision. Can use device.

   1: Needs help or supervision, but can perform

   0: Unable to perform

Dressing and undressing (0-2 points)

   2: Able to remove and put on all clothing,
       including shoes

   1: Needs help to put on or remove clothing
       in a reasonable time

   0: Unable to perform

Continence of bowel (0-2 points)

   2: Patient controls bowels. No accidents.
       Can use bedpan at bed rest.

   1: Occasionally incontinent

   0: Incontinent, no bowel control

Control of bladder (0-2 points)

   2: Controls bladder day and night.
       Can use bedpan at bed rest.

   1: Occasional accidents, needs help to void

   0: Unable to control bladder, frequently incontinent.
       Needs catheter.

mia,[9] or a consumption coagulopathy). For this reason, the blood smear must also be examined under the microscope. Polycythemia also can contribute to stroke.[10] The platelet count is necessary to establish hypercoagulability or a thrombotic disorder, such as thrombotic thrombocytopenic purpura[11] or idiopathic thrombocytic purpura,[12] which can lead to ischemic and hemorrhagic strokes. The white blood count is important to help identify infectious etiologies, such as endocarditis, or associated secondary infections such as pneumonia, as well as to rule out stroke associated with a hematologic malignancy, such as leukemia. Prothrombin time and partial thromboplastin time are necessary both to rule out a source of hemorrhage when they are elevated, and as a baseline for therapeutic interventions with anticoagulation or thrombolysis. Further coagulation studies, including anticardiolipin antibody,[13] protein C,[14] protein S,[15] and fibrinogen, which can increase blood viscosity,[16] often are obtained to identify hypercoagulability, particularly in younger patients with stroke.[17]

Chemical analysis of the blood is necessary to identify metabolic disorders that could contribute to the severity of the stroke, particularly hyperglycemia and hypoglycemia. In diabetics who present with focal neurologic deficits, a finger-stick glucose is appropriate because both hypoglycemia and nonketotic hyperosmolar hyperglycemia can present with focal neurologic deficits that are reversible by treating the glucose abnormality. Hyperglycemia may adversely affect the outcome of ischemic stroke, and should be rectified.[18] Hyponatremia can adversely affect stroke outcome by increasing cerebral edema. Calcium and potassium abnormalities can contribute to cardiac arrhythmias that can cause hypoperfusion of ischemic brain regions. Liver function and renal abnormalities can reduce the level of consciousness in a patient with stroke, which can lead to further complications. Elevated creatine phosphokinase (CPK) can indicate a concomitant myocardial infarction, al-

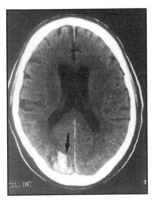

Figure 1: *Intracerebral hemorrhage. CT of the brain shows a white area (arrow) in the occipital lobe, representing blood. A small amount of lucent brain indicates surrounding edema. Immediate CT or MRI is necessary in the management of acute stroke before any antithrombotic treatment can be initiated, to be certain that the stroke is not from a cerebral hemorrhage. Figure courtesy of Dr. Adam Silvers.*

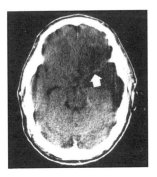

Figure 2: *CT of the brain shows a subacute infarct as a lucency in the middle cerebral artery territory extending from the frontal lobe to the temporal lobe and involving cortical and subcortical structures (white arrow). Figure courtesy of Dr. Adam Silvers.*

though serum CPK can also be elevated in a patient who has been lying immobile for a prolonged time, or may even arise directly from ischemic brain.

The EKG is critical to identify cardiac arrhythmias that may be the cause of the stroke or arise from the stroke, and become life-threatening. Atrial fibrillation is a major risk factor for stroke.[19] The presence of atrial fibrillation or flutter on the EKG suggests that the stroke is cardioembolic in origin, although other sources of stroke, such as carotid artery disease, can exist in the same patient.[20] Large ischemic strokes and hemorrhages also can produce inversion of T waves and U waves, as well as early repolarization, which can lead to ventricular fibrillation and torsades de pointes.[21,22] For this reason, hospitalizing stroke patients in a monitored bed, preferably in an acute stroke unit, often is desirable.

Neuroimaging Acute Stroke Patients

Imaging of the Brain

Radiographic CT is the most available and quickest method for imaging the brain in acute stroke patients.[23] With the advent of thrombolytic therapy, it is imperative to be able to immediately differentiate hemorrhagic from ischemic stroke; this can be done with CT. Hemorrhages appear as white densities almost as white as bone (Figure 1). Infarcts appear as lucencies relative to the density of the brain (Figure 2). In the acute phase of ischemic stroke, particularly in the first 3 hours, but sometimes up to 48 hours after onset of symptoms, no abnormalities may be seen on CT of the brain. In these instances, the examiner must rely on clinical examination to determine the type and severity of stroke when planning therapeutic decisions. Early changes of infarction, such as effacement of sulci and loss of clear-cut differentiation at the junction of the gray matter and white matter, sometimes can be seen, but this is often difficult to identify, even for experienced examiners.[24]

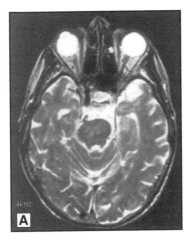

Figure 3: MRI of the brain performed on a patient within 6 hours of onset of an acute brain stem stroke. The T2 image (A) shows no evidence of infarction of the pons. A diffusion-weighted image of the pons (B) shows an area of infarction with diffusion of water into the region (arrow). Figure courtesy of Dr. Adam Silvers.

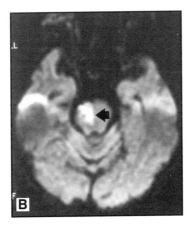

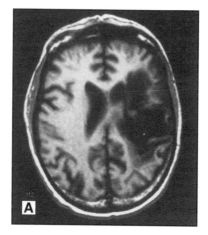

Figure 4: *MRI of the brain demonstrating an infarct in the middle cerebral artery with a T1-weighted image (A) and a T2-weighted image (B). Water is black in (A) and white in (B), as indicated by the shading of the ventricular system containing cerebrospinal fluid. An infarct in the distribution of an entire artery territory or branch is most often cardioembolic.* Courtesy of Dr. Adam Silvers.

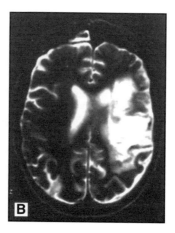

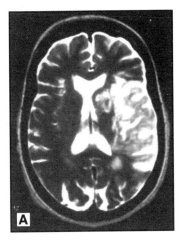

Figure 5: *(A) MRI of the brain shows an infarct in the middle cerebral artery territory on T2 imaging. A hemorrhagic component occurs in the region of the basal ganglia next to the lateral ventricle. (B) The area of hemorrhage can be seen as a dark spot in the diffusion-weighted image and gradient echo image of the infarct (C) (arrow).* Figure courtesy of Dr. Adam Silvers.

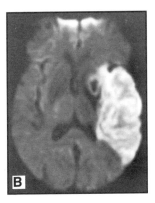

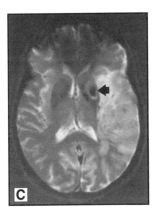

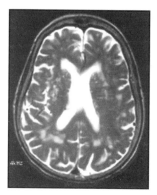

Figure 6: Multiple areas of ischemia (white) are seen on a T2-weighted MRI of a patient with an acute stroke. This is the pattern seen with thrombosis of small intracranial vessels secondary to diabetes and hypertension. Figure courtesy of Dr. Adam Silvers.

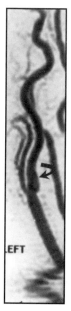

Figure 7: MRA of a normal carotid artery bifurcation. Figure courtesy of Dr. Adam Silvers.

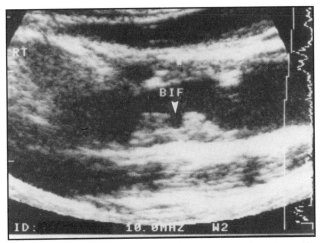

Figure 8: Real-time B-mode ultrasonography of an atherosclerotic plaque in the carotid artery bifurcation, causing a stenosis. From Weinberger J, Tegeler CH, McKinney WM, et al: Ultrasonography for diagnosis and management of carotid artery atherosclerosis. A position paper of the American Society of Neuroimaging. J Neuroimaging 1995;5:237-243.

Changes of cerebral infarction are seen earlier with MRI than with CT,[25] particularly with the new technique of diffusion MRI, which measures regions of diffusing brain water into ischemic areas[26] (Figure 3). However, even these techniques may not visualize the extent and location of the infarction for several hours after onset of ischemia.

Imaging of the brain can also aid in determining stroke subtype. When an infarct involving the cortex in the discrete distribution of a particular artery is identified, the stroke is more likely attributable to a cardioembolic mechanism (Figure 4). A hemorrhagic component to the infarct also suggests a cardioembolic source, because hem-

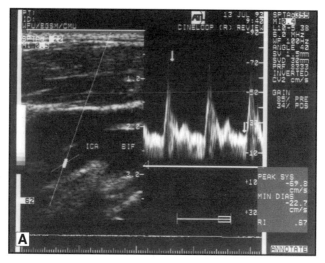

Figure 9: Spectral analysis of Doppler ultrasound frequency shifts. (A) Normal internal carotid artery flow velocity; (B) Elevated flow velocity in systole and diastole with high-grade internal carotid artery stenosis. From Weinberger J, et al, as in Figure 8.

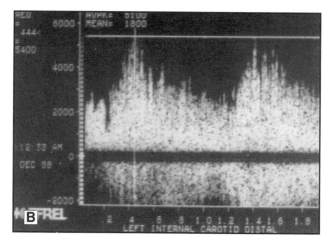

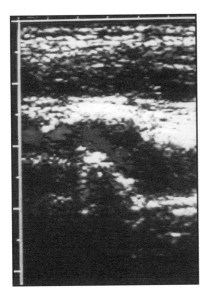

Figure 10: Color flow duplex Doppler sonography outlines the carotid artery bifurcation. From Weinberger J, et al, as in Figure 8.

orrhage often develops with reperfusion of the infarcted brain after lysis of the embolic thrombus (Figure 5).[27] Lacunar infarcts from small-vessel intracranial thrombosis may not be visualized on CT, but are detected as bright spots on MRI, mainly in the periventricular regions of the white matter (Figure 6). The blood vessels to the brain that may be responsible for the stroke also can be imaged by MRI with MRA (Figure 7) and by CT angiography.

Noninvasive ultrasound techniques employ B-mode imaging to visualize atherosclerotic plaque in the extracranial carotid bifurcation[28] (Figure 8), and measure flow in the extracranial[29] and intracranial vessels[30] with Doppler ultrasound. Doppler measures the velocity of blood flow by emitting an ultrasound beam, 5 to 10 MHz, which is reflected back to the transducer by the flowing red blood cells. The frequency of the echo shifts into the audible range of sound, which can be plotted by spectral analysis of frequencies with a fast Fourrier transform (Figure 9).

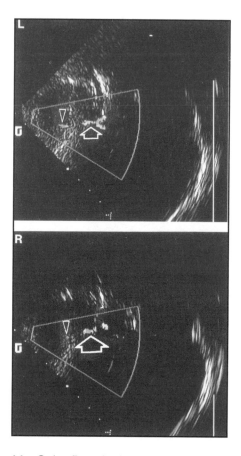

Figure 11: Color flow duplex sonography of a normal middle cerebral artery (L) and a stenotic middle cerebral artery (R). The trunk of the middle cerebral artery is indicated by a large arrow, and the region of the stenosis in the distal middle cerebral artery is indicated by the caret. From Weinberger J, et al: Identification of stenosis of the opercular segment of the middle cerebral artery trunk by transcranial color flow duplex Doppler. J Stroke Cerebrovasc Dis 1992;2:209-212.

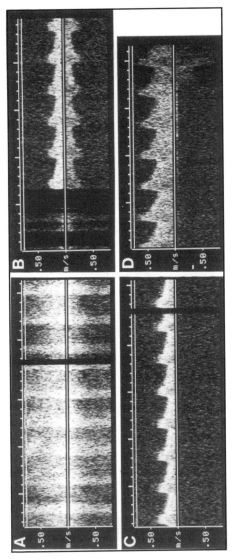

Figure 12: *Spectral frequency shift analysis of Doppler velocities in the middle cerebral artery. Panel A shows elevation of flow velocity with spread of frequencies in the region of the stenosis. Panel B shows reduction of flow proximal to the stenosis with a retrograde component. Panel C shows the normal flow in the distal middle cerebral artery in the same region as the stenosis on the normal contralateral side. Panel D shows the normal flow pattern in the contralateral middle cerebral artery trunk. From Weinberger J, et al, as in Figure 11.*

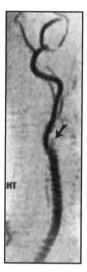

Figure 13: *A complete occlusion of the internal carotid artery is seen with MRA imaging. The stump of the internal carotid can be visualized. Occasionally, in low-flow states, both Doppler and MRA may not detect a trickle of flow at the site of what appears to be the occlusion but, in this case, reconstitution of the internal carotid artery should be seen distally.* Figure courtesy of Dr. Adam Silvers.

The frequency shift is proportional to the velocity of the flowing red cells, and velocity can be calculated if the angle of insonation is known. Velocity is elevated in areas of stenosis of the artery and is proportional to the residual lumen area, so the accuracy of the Doppler technique may more reflect the hemodynamics of the stenosis than angiography and MRA.[31] The vessel can be imaged in color with Doppler by assigning red to flow directed toward the probe, and blue to flow directed away from the probe, with yellow indicating stenosis by assigning this color to all velocities over a critical threshold (Figure 10). However, frequency shift analysis is still necessary to quantify the degree of stenosis, even when it can be visualized in color flow.

Doppler ultrasound can also be used to measure flow velocity in the intracranial vessels[32] and image the arteries with color flow duplex Doppler (Figure 11).[33] A low-

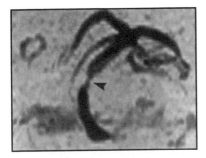

Figure 14: *MRA of a basilar artery stenosis (arrow). Figure courtesy of Dr. Adam Silvers.*

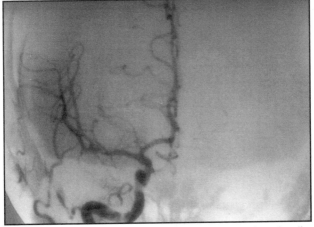

Figure 15: *Intra-arterial contrast angiography of a distal middle cerebral artery stenosis just proximal to the vertical takeoff of the middle cerebral artery branches. This angiogram is from the same patient in whom middle cerebral artery stenosis was detected by transcranial Doppler sonography in Figures 11 and 12. From Weinberger J, et al, as in Figure 11.*

frequency, 2-MHz Doppler probe is employed to penetrate thin sections of bone. The middle cerebral and anterior cerebral arteries are insonated through the anterior transtemporal window, and the posterior cerebral arteries are insonated through the posterior temporal window about the level of the external auditory meatus. The ophthalmic artery, and intracranial internal carotid artery as it passes through the cavernous sinus, can be measured through the orbit (lowering the power of the transducer to 10%). The vertebral and basilar arteries are insonated through the foramen magnum on each side just below the ear. The distance from the probe in millimeters and the direction of flow toward or away from the probe identify the vessel being insonated. Stenosis is identified by elevation of velocity (Figure 12).

Transcranial Doppler can also be used to assess collateral circulation and intracranial hemodynamics in patients with carotid occlusive disease. Retrograde flow through the ophthalmic artery, or cross-filling through the anterior communicating artery to feed the anterior cerebral artery ipsilateral to a lesion at the carotid artery bifurcation, indicates hemodynamically significant stenosis because of that good collateral flow. If collateral flow is not present, but flow velocity in the ipsilateral middle cerebral artery is reduced with decreased pulsatility, a hemodynamic stenosis without good collateral flow is present.[34]

MRI can visualize the extracranial (Figure 13) and intracranial (Figure 14) arteries noninvasively, using a subtraction technique to outline the void in the signal created by flowing blood.[35] An image of the artery is formed that appears similar to the image produced by intra-arterial contrast angiography, but the image depends on flow velocity, and does not exactly represent the walls and lumen of the artery. CT angiography does show an anatomic outline of the arteries, but requires injection of contrast, which introduces the risk of allergic reaction or fluid overload in elderly patients with congestive heart failure. Angiography with intra-arterial injection of contrast dye is still considered the gold standard for demonstrating vascular lesions (Figure 15).

Echocardiography also is obtained in most stroke patients to document a cardioembolic source of stroke. The accuracy of finding thrombus in the left atrium is greatly increased by transesophageal echocardiography (TEE)[36] (Figure 16). Atheroma in the arch of the aorta has been implicated as a source of cerebral thromboembolism, and these can be visualized by TEE (Figure 17), although transcutaneous B-mode imaging of the aortic arch also can identify aortic arch atheroma.[37] Shunting of blood from the right to the left atrium through a patent foramen ovale or atrial septal defect can allow thrombus from the peripheral veins to pass through the arterial circulation and occlude cerebral arteries without being filtered by the lungs.[38] These right-to-left shunts can be visualized by TEE with injection of contrast bubbles, which can be seen passing from the right atrium to the left atrium (Figure 18).

Imaging Cerebral Blood Flow

Blood flow to the brain can be measured by a variety of techniques. The most readily available method is SPECT. SPECT uses a nuclear isotope, usually technetium Tc 99m-labeled HMPAO[38] or inhaled or intravenous xenon Xe 133,[39] which emits a single photon that can be detected by a ring of transducers to provide a tomographic image of the brain, similar to CT. The isotope distributes in the regions of blood flow and can show perfusion deficits in stroke in areas that may not show infarction on CT or MRI (Figure 19). Technetium Tc 99 HMPAO or iodine I 123 iodoamphetamine provides an image of perfusion, while measuring xenon Xe 133 washout can actually quantify blood flow expressed in mL/100 g/minute in different regions of brain. Nonradioactive xenon also can image perfusion by injecting xenon intravenously during CT of the brain, and can be quantified by measuring the time of washout of the xenon as well.[40] Perfusion-weighted imaging can make a similar image of blood flow on MRI, but cannot quanti-

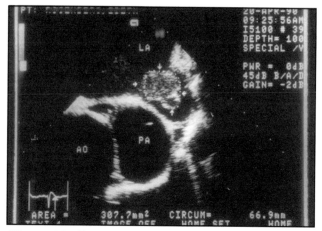

Figure 16: *Transesophageal echocardiography of a thrombus in the left atrium of a patient with a cardioembolic stroke. Figure courtesy of Dr. Martin Goldman.*

fy the rate of flow.[41] PET employs isotopes that emit two photons at 180 degrees. A ring detector can identify the location of the isotope much more precisely than SPECT, providing a resolution down to 5 mm.[42] Blood flow can be measured by inhalation of oxygen O 15-labeled carbon dioxide or nitrogen N 13-labeled ammonia, which dissolves in the blood and distributes with cerebral blood flow. The rate of oxygen use and oxygen extraction fraction can define cerebral metabolism and oxygen extraction in different regions of brain to identify areas of hypometabolism and vulnerable brain tissue. Regional brain glucose metabolic rate can be measured with 2 (18F)-fluorodeoxyglucose to identify hypometabolic regions, which also can image regional increases in brain metabolism during mental activities or tasks to provide images of regional brain function. Positron-labeled receptor ligands can also be imaged to study regional neuro-

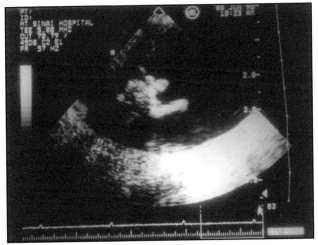

Figure 17: *Transesophageal echocardiography of an atherosclerotic plaque with thrombus in the aortic arch of a patient with stroke. From Weinberger J: Current management strategies for cerebrovascular stenosis: prophylaxis and treatment. In: Peterson PL, Phillis JW: Novel Therapies for CNS Injuries. Rationales and Results. Boca Raton, Fla, CRC Press, 1995, pp 69-90. Figure courtesy of Dr. Martin Goldman.*

pharmacology. Although PET has opened broad areas of research into the mechanisms of brain function, it is not readily applicable to management of stroke patients because of its expense and complexity.

The Diagnosis of Stroke

The findings of the clinical examination, and imaging of the brain, extracranial and intracranial arteries, and the heart, must be examined to determine the type of stroke. This determines treatment to prevent further strokes and worsening of the current stroke. With the advent of new treatments that can reduce the amount of neurologic deficit and disability

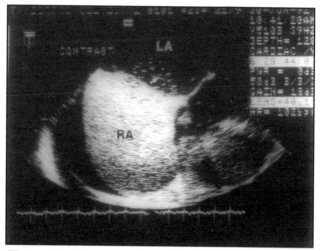

Figure 18: *Transesophageal echocardiography demonstrating contrast bubbles flow from the right atrium (RA) to the left atrium (LA) in a patient with stroke who had a patent foramen ovale. From Weinberger J, as in Figure 17. Figure courtesy of Dr. Martin Goldman.*

when applied within 3 hours, immediate identification of the etiology of the stroke becomes crucial.

Although history and clinical examination are still the best early indicators of stroke severity, location, and subtype, emergency imaging of the brain is necessary to differentiate ischemic stroke from hemorrhage. If MRI is used to image the brain, MRA of the extracranial and intracranial vessels can be performed at the same time. If CT is performed, CT angiography can be performed at the same time. Doppler ultrasound studies can be used at the bedside as part of the clinical examination to identify occlusive disease of the intracranial and extracranial vasculature. The entire diagnostic evaluation must be completed in sufficient time so that therapy can be instituted within 3 hours of onset of symptoms if treatment is indicated.

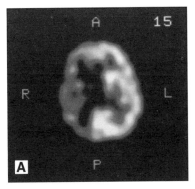

Figure 19: SPECT shows decreased cerebral perfusion of the entire right hemisphere (A) in a patient with a left hemiplegia. CT of the brain showed only a small right basal ganglia infarction, even 72 hours after the stroke (B). From Weinberger J: The significance of basal ganglia infarction. J Stroke Cerebrovasc Dis *1995;5:6-11.*

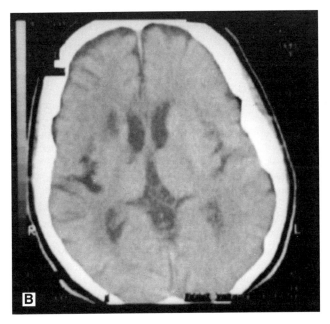

References

1. Bogousslavsky J, Van Melle G, Regli F: The Lausanne Stroke Registry: analysis of 1,000 consecutive patients with first stroke. *Stroke* 1988;19:1083-1092.

2. Gordon DL, Bendixen BH, Adams HP Jr, et al: Interphysician agreement in the diagnosis of subtypes of acute ischemic stroke: implications for clinical trials. The TOAST Investigators. *Neurology* 1993;43:1021-1027.

3. Lhermitte F, Gautier JC, Derouesne C: Nature of occlusions of the middle cerebral artery. *Neurology* 1970;20:82-88.

4. Fisher CM: Lacunes: small deep cerebral infarcts. *Neurology* 1965;15:774-778.

5. Brott T, Adams HP Jr, Olinger CP, et al: Measurements of acute cerebral infarction: a clinical examination scale. *Stroke* 1989;20:864-870.

6. Teasdale G, Jennett B: Assessment of coma and impaired consciousness. A practical scale. *Lancet* 1974;2:81-84.

7. Mahoney FI, Barthel DW: Functional evaluation. The Barthel Index. *Maryland St Med J* 1965;14:61-65.

8. The National Institute of Neurological Disorders and Stroke rt-PA Stroke Study Group: Tissue plasminogen activator for acute ischemic stroke. *N Engl J Med* 1995;333:1581-1587.

9. Russell MO, Goldberg HI, Hodson A, et al: Effect of transfusion therapy on arteriographic abnormalities and on recurrence of stroke in sickle cell disease. *Blood* 1984;63:162-169.

10. Kannel WB, Gordon T, Wolf PA, et al: Hemoglobin and the risk of cerebral infarction: the Framingham Study. *Stroke* 1972;3:409-420.

11. Silverstein A: Thrombotic thrombocytopenic purpura. The initial neurologic manifestations. *Arch Neurol* 1968;18:358-362.

12. DiFino SM, Lachant NA, Kirshner JJ, et al: Adult idiopathic thrombocytopenic purpura. Clinical findings and response to therapy. *Am J Med* 1980;69:430-442.

13. The Antiphospholipid Antibodies in Stroke Study (APASS) Group: Anticardiolipin antibodies are an independent risk factor for first ischemic stroke. *Neurology* 1993;43:2069-2073.

14. D'Angelo A, Vigano-D'Angelo S, Esmon CT, et al: Acquired deficiencies of protein S. Protein S activity during oral anticoagu-

lation, in liver disease, and in disseminated intravascular coagulation. *J Clin Invest* 1988;81:1445-1454.

15. Kohler J, Kasper J, Witt L, et al: Ischemic stroke due to protein C deficiency. *Stroke* 1990;21:1077-1080.

16. Shanker R, Fisher M: Fibrinogen and stroke. In: Adams HP Jr: *Handbook of Cerebrovascular Diseases*. New York, Marcel Dekker, 1993, pp 1-12.

17. Hart RG, Miller VT: Cerebral infarction in young adults: a practical approach. *Stroke* 1983;14:110-114.

18. Woo J, Lam CW, Kay R, et al: The influence of hyperglycemia and diabetes mellitus on immediate and 3-month morbidity and mortality after acute stroke. *Arch Neurol* 1990; 47:1174-1177.

19. Wolf PA, Dawber TR, Thomas HE Jr, et al: Epidemiologic assessment of chronic atrial fibrillation and risk of stroke: the Framingham Study. *Neurology* 1978;28:973-977.

20. Weinberger J, Rothlauf E, Materese E, et al: Noninvasive evaluation of the extracranial carotid arteries in patients with cerebrovascular events and atrial fibrillations. *Arch Intern Med* 1988; 148:1785-1788.

21. Dimant J, Grob D: Electrocardiographic changes and myocardial damage in patients with acute cerebrovascular accidents. *Stroke* 1977;8:448-455.

22. Mikolich JR, Jacobs WC, Fletcher GF: Cardiac arrhythmias in patients with acute cerebrovascular accidents. *JAMA* 1981; 246:1314-1317.

23. Culebras A, Kase CS, Masdeu JC, et al: Practice guidelines for the use of imaging in transient ischemic attacks and acute stroke. A report of the Stroke Council, American Heart Association. *Stroke* 1997;28:1480-1497.

24. Larrue V, von Kummer R, del Zoppo G, et al: Hemorrhagic transformation in acute ischemic stroke. Potential contributing factors in the European Cooperative Acute Stroke Study. *Stroke* 1997;28:957-960.

25. DeWitt LD: Clinical use of nuclear magnetic resonance imaging in stroke. *Stroke* 1986;17:328-331.

26. Warach S, Gaa J, Siewert B, et al: Acute human stroke studied by whole brain echo planar diffusion-weighted MRI. *Ann Neurol* 1995;37:231-241.

27. Ramirez-Lassepas M, Quinones MR: Heparin therapy for stroke: hemorrhagic complications and risk factors for intracerebral hemorrhage. *Neurology* 1984;34:114-117.

28. Weinberger J, Robbins A: Neurologic symptoms associated with nonobstructive plaque at carotid bifurcation. Analysis by real-time B-mode ultrasonography. *Arch Neurol* 1983;40:489-492.

29. Blackshear WM Jr, Phillips DJ, Thiele BL, et al: Detection of carotid occlusive disease by ultrasonic imaging and pulsed Doppler spectrum analysis. *Surgery* 1979;86:698-706.

30. Aaslid R, Markwalder TM, Nornes H: Noninvasive transcranial Doppler ultrasound recording of flow velocity in basal cerebral arteries. *J Neurosurg* 1982;57:769-774.

31. Suwanwela N, Can U, Furie KL, et al: Carotid Doppler ultrasound criteria for internal carotid artery stenosis based on residual lumen diameter calculated from en bloc carotid endarterectomy specimens. *Stroke* 1996;27:1965-1969.

32. Ringelstein EB: A practical guide to transcranial Doppler sonography. In: Weinberger J: *Noninvasive Imaging of the Cerebral Circulation. Frontiers of Clinical Neuroscience*, Vol. 5. New York, Alan R. Liss, 1989, pp 75-123.

33. Bogdahn U, Becker G, Winkler J, et al: Transcranial color-coded real-time sonography in adults. *Stroke* 1990;21:1680-1688.

34. Wilterdink JL, Feldmann E, Furie KL, et al: Transcranial Doppler ultrasound battery reliably identifies severe internal carotid artery stenosis. *Stroke* 1997;28:133-136.

35. Ruszkowski JT, Damadian R, Giambalvo A, et al: MRI angiography of the carotid artery. *Magn Reson Imaging* 1986;4:497-502.

36. Horowitz DR, Tuhrim S, Weinberger J, et al: Transesophageal echocardiography: diagnostic and clinical applications in the evaluation of the stroke patient. *J Stroke Cerebrovasc Dis* 1997;6:332-336.

37. Weinberger J, Azhar S, Danisi F, et al: A new noninvasive technique for imaging atherosclerotic plaque in the aortic arch of stroke patients by transcutaneous real-time B-mode ultrasonography: an initial report. *Stroke* 1998;29:673-676.

38. Holman BL, Moretti JL, Hill TC: SPECT perfusion imaging in cerebrovascular disease. In: Weinberger J: *Noninvasive Imag-*

ing of *Cerebrovascular Disease. Frontiers of Clinical Neuroscience*, Vol. 5. New York, Alan R. Liss, 1989, pp 147-162.

39. Obrist WD, Thompson HK Jr, Wang HS, et al: Regional cerebral blood flow estimated by 133-xenon inhalation. *Stroke* 1975; 6:245-256.

40. Johnson DW, Stringer WA, Marks MP, et al: Stable xenon CT cerebral blood flow imaging: rationale for and role in clinical decision making. *Am J Neuroradiol* 1991;12:201-213.

41. Warach S, Dashe JF, Edelman RR: Clinical outcome in ischemic stroke predicted by early diffusion-weighted and perfusion magnetic resonance imaging: a preliminary analysis. *J Cereb Blood Flow Metab* 1996;16:53-59.

42. Kushner M, Reivich M: Functional imaging of brain ischemia. In: Weinberger J: *Noninvasive Imaging of Cerebrovascular Disease. Frontiers of Clinical Neuroscience*, Vol. 5. New York, Alan R. Liss, 1989, pp 163-174.

Chapter **3**

Primary Prevention of Stroke

A recent advance in the treatment of acute stroke has created considerable excitement. That advance is thrombolytic therapy with tissue plasminogen activator, which has proved beneficial in improving outcome when administered within 3 hours of onset.[1] Nevertheless, the prevention of cerebrovascular disease leading to stroke is still the optimal goal for reducing the morbidity and disability associated with this devastating illness. The strategy for primary prevention of stroke is to address the major risk factors for cerebrovascular disease (Table 1): hypertension; diabetes; metabolic and nutritional disorders leading to atherosclerosis; smoking; and cardiogenic emboli, particularly from atrial fibrillation.

Hypertension

Hypertension is the most important risk factor for ischemic stroke.[2] It has been documented since the 1960s that even a blood pressure of 130/90 in young males 30 to 40 years old is considered hypertension. Antihypertensive treatment reduces the stroke rate by 50% in these patients.[3-6] However, it is not clear that the treatment of hypertension in young and middle-aged women is effective in preventing stroke.[7] A recent meta-analysis demonstrated that treatment of hypertension with beta-blockers or hydrochlorothiazide diuretics is equally effective in pre-

Table 1: Control of Risk Factors

Hypertension	Blood pressure reduction
Diabetes	Control of blood sugar
Atherosclerosis	Reduction of elevated LDL cholesterol
	Drug therapy: pravastatin, simvastatin
	Vitamin supplementation: vitamin E, beta carotene, vitamin B_6, vitamin B_{12}, folic acid
	Estrogen replacement therapy in women
	Platelet antiaggregant therapy: aspirin, clopidogrel, ticlopidine
	Cessation of smoking
	Identification and treatment of asymptomatic carotid stenosis
Cardiogenic emboli	Identification and treatment of nonvalvular atrial fibrillation
	• Low risk: aspirin
	• High risk: warfarin INR 3.0 to 3.5
	• Over age 75: warfarin INR range 2.0 to 2.5
	Rheumatic valve disease and atrial fibrillation, valve replacement
	• Warfarin INR range 2.8 to 3.5
	Post-myocardial infarction
	• Warfarin INR range 2.5 to 3.0 for 3 months

venting stroke in women as in men.[8] Treatment of hypertension in the elderly, including isolated systolic hypertension, also has been controversial, but has been effective in preventing stroke.[9,10] The Systolic Hypertension in the Elderly Program showed reduction in the incidence of stroke with a thiazide-class diuretic.[9] The Systolic Hypertension in Europe Trial demonstrated a reduction in incidence of stroke with a long-acting calcium-channel blocker, nitrendipine.[10] Therefore, treatment of hypertension in all age groups and genders appears to be effective in reducing the risk of stroke.

Evidence suggests that calcium-channel blockers, particularly the short-acting nifedipine preparation (Adalat®, Procardia®), may increase the risk of myocardial infarction compared with the other classes, such as beta-blockers and angiotensin-converting enzyme (ACE) inhibitors.[11-14] The results should be available soon of a trial (ALLHAT) of the antihypertensive agents amlodipine (Norvasc®), a long-acting calcium-channel blocker; lisinopril, an ACE inhibitor; and doxazosin (Cardura®), an alpha-adrenergic receptor blocker, in combination with the diuretic chlorthalidone in hypertensive patients more than 55 years old.[11,15] This study will document whether these other antihypertensive agents are as effective as calcium-channel blockers, beta-adrenergic blockers, and thiazide-type diuretics in preventing stroke in the elderly, as well as whether amlodipine can be safely used to prevent stroke without increasing the risk of myocardial infarction.

Diabetes

Diabetes is another major risk factor for stroke.[16] Diabetes produces proliferative changes of the walls of small intracranial vessels, resulting in thrombosis, and promotes atherosclerosis of large intracranial and extracranial arteries.[17,18] Diabetes also causes platelet hyperaggregability and serum hypercoagulability, which can cause thrombosis of stenotic arteries.[19] Hyperglycemia increases the extent of brain injury during ischemia,[20,21] and contributes to the risk of stroke regardless of the extent of extracranial vascular disease because of its direct effects on cerebral blood flow and metabolism.[22]

Although it has never been established that strict control of blood sugar in diabetics prevents ischemic stroke, it can lessen the degree of proliferative small-artery vascular changes in the retina,[23] and may be able to prevent these changes in cerebral vessels as well. Diabetes is the greatest predictor of mortality during ischemic stroke,[24] suggesting that effective control of glucose is beneficial for prevention of stroke as well as for outcome after stroke.

Serum Lipids and Atherosclerosis

Elevation of serum cholesterol has been established as one of the most significant risk factors for coronary artery disease, but the same relationship has not been established for ischemic stroke.[25] This may partly result from the differential etiologies of ischemic stroke. In a study of Japanese men adjusted for age and hypertension, patients with stroke from large-vessel atherosclerotic disease had an increased serum total cholesterol (mean 200 mg/dL), but patients with stroke from occlusion of small penetrating vessels had a low serum total cholesterol (mean 177 mg/dL).[26] Low cholesterol appeared to be associated with the arteriolar necrosis and lipohyalinization of small vessels responsible for intracranial thrombosis.[26] Therefore, reducing cholesterol may prevent atherosclerotic cerebrovascular disease, but could contribute to cerebrovascular disease in patients with intracranial arteriolar vasculopathy.

Reduction of lipids in dietary intake has been beneficial in preventing coronary artery disease, but the risk of stroke is reduced in patients with an adequate intake of saturated and monounsaturated fats, while there was no relationship to the intake of polyunsaturated fats.[27] The results of this study raised the possibility that restriction of fat intake does not decrease and could increase the overall risk of ischemic stroke.[27]

Other dietary factors may be involved in a reduction in the incidence of stroke from atherosclerosis. Fish consumption at least once a week in white women and African-American men and women reduced the incidence of stroke by 50%, though fish consumption and stroke risk were not associated in white men.[28] High dietary contents of the antioxidants beta carotene and vitamin E also have been shown to reduce the incidence of stroke, probably by stabilizing atherosclerotic plaques to prevent propagation.[29,30]

Homocysteine has been found to be elevated to plasma concentrations of 20 to 40 µmol/L in patients with cerebrovascular disease.[31] While the normal range for homocysteine is 5 to 15 µmol/L, atherosclerosis is increased in the carotid artery with plasma concentrations as low as 11.4 to 14.3 µmol/L. Homocysteine is metabolized to methionine with enzymes requiring vitamin B_{12} and folic acid, and to cystathionine with enzymes requiring vitamin B_6. Increasing intake of folic acid by 200 µg/d can reduce plasma homocysteine concentration by 4 µmol/L, and thus significantly reduce the risk of vascular disease.[31] Although a prospective study is needed to document that lowering plasma homocysteine concentration reduces the incidence of stroke, adequate dietary intake of folic acid, vitamin B_{12}, and vitamin B_6 should be encouraged, particularly in patients with plasma levels of homocysteine greater than 15 µmol/L.

Although dietary reduction of lipid intake in the general population may not help prevent stroke, treatment of patients with coronary artery disease or elevated cholesterol has been remarkably successful in preventing ischemic stroke.[32] Two members of a new class of cholesterol-lowering agents, 3-hydroxy-3-methylglutaryl coenzyme A (HMG CoA) reductase inhibitors, have been shown to lower the risk of recurrent myocardial infarction and CHD death in patients with symptomatic coronary artery disease.[33-36] In addition, these two agents, simvastatin (Zocor®) and pravastatin (Pravachol®), have been shown to reduce the incidence of stroke and TIA in patients with established CHD.[35-37] This reduction in stroke occurs in patients with elevated cholesterol and in those with normal cholesterol.[38,39] These patients are more likely to develop large-vessel atherosclerotic cerebrovascular disease. Reduction of LDL cholesterol with lovastatin (Mevacor®) and pravastatin decreased the degree of carotid artery atherosclerosis when intimal-medial thickness (IMT) was measured with B-mode sonography.[40,41]

Antithrombotic therapy with the platelet antiaggregant aspirin has been effective in reducing events associated with coronary artery disease, but has shown no benefit in preventing stroke in patients not at direct risk for cerebrovascular disease.[42] In both the Physicians' Health Study and the International Study of Infarct Survival, aspirin therapy prevented myocardial infarction, but not ischemic stroke.[43,44]

The new platelet antiaggregant agent clopidogrel (Plavix®) 75 mg q.d. has been shown to have an 8.7% improved risk reduction over aspirin 325 mg q.d. for preventing the combined ischemic events of stroke, myocardial infarction, and vascular death in patients with preexisting atherosclerotic disease manifested by recent ischemic stroke, established peripheral vascular disease, or recent myocardial infarction.[45] The study population consisted of 19,185 patients, 12,200 of whom had not had a previous ischemic stroke. Extrapolation from these data may be valid that for patients who have atherosclerotic disease and who are asymptomatic for stroke, treatment with clopidogrel may help prevent first stroke.

Smoking

Cigarette smoking, as measured by nicotine excretion, has been shown to increase IMT in the carotid artery. It is an independent risk factor for stroke.[46] Cessation of smoking reduces IMT in the carotid artery, and lessens the propagation of atherosclerosis in carotid artery plaques.[46,47] Cessation of smoking appears beneficial in preventing large-vessel atherosclerotic cerebrovascular disease.

Hormonal Status in Women

Women of child-bearing age have a low rate of ischemic stroke, which is not increased during pregnancy.[48,49] However, the relative risk of stroke is increased 2.4 times during the puerperium, for up to 6 weeks after the pregnancy.[50] The factors responsible for this increase in stroke have not been clarified. The use of oral contraceptives slightly increases the risk of stroke, and they can be used safely in women under age 35 who do not smoke and who are not hypertensive.[50] In postmenopausal women, estrogen and estrogen/progesterone replacement therapy often are used to reduce coronary artery disease. Both estrogen and estrogen/progesterone decrease the degree of carotid artery IMT, and appear beneficial in preventing cerebrovascular disease.[51]

Asymptomatic Carotid Artery Stenosis

Patients with asymptomatic atherosclerosis of the extra-cranial carotid artery bifurcation are often identified by the auscultation of a vascular bruit on the neck.[52] These patients usually are screened with carotid duplex sonography to determine the presence of a carotid artery stenosis, and the degree of obstruction to flow. Doppler frequency shift analysis provides a measure of lumen diameter reduction compared to angiography,[53] and area reduction compared to pathologic specimens,[54] with an accuracy of 95%.

The management of asymptomatic carotid artery stenosis remains controversial. Carotid endarterectomy has been shown to have some value in patients with greater than 60% diameter reduction of the internal carotid artery documented by intra-arterial contrast angiography, but the out-

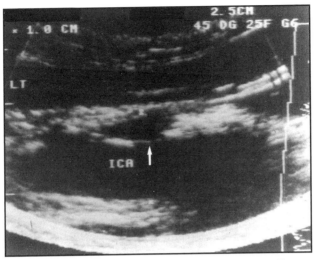

Figure 1: *A heterogeneous plaque with a thin fibrous cap in the carotid artery bifurcation seen with real-time B-mode ultrasonography. The lucent area under the fibrous cap contains lipid and thrombus. These lesions are prone to rupture, producing symptoms of transient ischemic attack and stroke.[61] Used with permission.*

come of the surgical group was only slightly better than the outcome of the medical group treated with aspirin. The Asymptomatic Carotid Atherosclerosis Study (ACAS) demonstrated a 10% risk of stroke in the medical group treated with aspirin 650 mg b.i.d., compared with a 5% risk of stroke in the surgically treated group over a 5-year follow-up.[55] Although the risk reduction was calculated as 50%, the overall reduction in the incidence of stroke was 5%, and the results did not diverge until the fifth year of follow-up. Furthermore, endarterectomy had no beneficial effect in women.

Duplex Doppler sonography has been used to identify patients with asymptomatic carotid artery stenosis

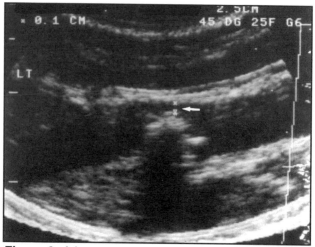

Figure 2: *A homogeneous plaque in the carotid artery bifurcation seen with real-time B-mode ultrasonography. The plaque is uniformly echodense, indicating that it contains fibrous and calcified plaque without thrombus, which is less likely to cause symptoms of transient ischemic attack or stroke.*

who are more likely at high risk of stroke, and would derive more benefit from carotid endarterectomy. Patients with progressive stenosis to 80% diameter reduction,[56] and patients with growth of plaque over time,[57] are more likely to become symptomatic than are patients with chronic static lesions. Patients with heterogeneous lucencies visualized with B-mode sonography within the plaque are at significantly greater risk of ipsilateral ischemic symptoms,[58] and of developing ipsilateral ischemic symptoms.[59,60] Therefore, in some centers, asymptomatic patients with greater than 60% stenosis of the internal carotid artery are referred for carotid endarterectomy if surgery is not contraindicated by coexisting medical conditions. The remainder are followed with sequential duplex Doppler sonography to identify progression or development of heterogeneous changes (Figures 1 and 2), at which point surgery may become indicated.[61] These patients are generally treated with aspirin for antithrombotic therapy, although whether patients with asymptomatic carotid stenosis fare better with aspirin therapy than with placebo has not been investigated.

Before performing carotid endarterectomy, magnetic resonance angiography of the carotid artery bifurcation is usually performed to confirm the Doppler findings, and to provide the surgeon with a more familiar view of the carotid bifurcation. The two studies are complementary and, in combination, provide an accurate estimate of the percent stenosis very close to intra-arterial contrast angiography, without the risk of catheterization.[62] When the two studies do not agree, contrast angiography becomes necessary to determine which result is correct.[61]

Patients undergoing coronary bypass surgery, peripheral vascular surgery, or abdominal vascular surgery have a 15% coincidence of significant asymptomatic carotid artery stenosis, and are at risk for stroke during these complicated vascular procedures.[63-65] However, the incidence of stroke and degree of carotid stenosis have not been correlated during these procedures, and prophylactic carotid endarterectomy before vascular or cardiac surgery has not proven effective in preventing the risk of stroke.[63-65]

Prevention of Cardioembolic Stroke

The greatest risk factor for cardioembolic stroke, particularly in the elderly, is nonvalvular atrial fibrillation. It carries a risk of stroke of about 5% a year when untreated.[66] Anticoagulation with warfarin (Coumadin®) provides a 70% risk reduction of stroke for these patients, while aspirin only provides a 20% risk reduction.[67] Patients under 70 with atrial fibrillation but no other associated heart disease can be effectively managed with aspirin to prevent strokes.[68,69]

Patients under 70 with associated cardiac disease, such as congestive heart failure or left ventricular hypertrophy, are at higher risk for embolic stroke while on aspirin therapy.[70,71] These patients are generally treated with warfarin for stroke prophylaxis.

In patients over 70 with atrial fibrillation, all clinical trials have shown that warfarin is effective in preventing ischemic stroke, while aspirin is ineffective.[68,69,72-74] However, in patients over 75, the risk of hemorrhagic complications is significant, which negated the protective effect of warfarin against ischemic stroke in the Stroke Prevention in Atrial Fibrillation (SPAF) Trial.[69] However, the degree of anticoagulation in the SPAF Trial as measured by the international normalized ratio (INR) was higher than in the other trials of warfarin to prevent stroke such that, when results were pooled, the benefit of anticoagulation with warfarin in the elderly was significant.[67] Therefore, the recommendation is to treat patients over 75 with nonvalvular atrial fibrillation with warfarin for stroke prophylaxis, keeping the INR between 2.0 and 2.9, with a target of 2.5.[67]

Patients with atrial fibrillation and mitral stenosis, and patients with mechanical cardiac valve replacements, are generally treated with warfarin for prevention of embolic stroke, with the INR maintained between 3.0 to 3.5.[75] Anticoagulation with warfarin has also been beneficial in preventing stroke during the first 3 months after myocardial infarction, and is particularly useful in patients with large anterior wall infarction and akinetic wall segments.[76]

Conclusion

The major risk factors for stroke are well known, and strategies based on these risk factors for primary prevention of stroke are available. Nevertheless, stroke continues to be the third leading cause of death and the chief cause of disability in the United States. The mission of primary care physicians is to identify patients at risk for stroke, to recommend appropriate preventive therapy, and to ensure patient compliance with the treatment regimen. Aggressive management of patients at risk for stroke should have a significant impact on reducing the incidence of this debilitating disease.

References

1. The National Institute of Neurological Disorders and Stroke rt-PA Stroke Study Group: Tissue plasminogen activator for acute ischemic stroke. *N Engl J Med* 1995;333:1581-1587.

2. Kannel WB, Dawber TR, Sorlie P, et al: Components of blood pressure and risk of atherothrombotic brain infarction: the Framingham Study. *Stroke* 1976;7:327-331.

3. Hypertension-Stroke Cooperative Study Group: Effect of antihypertensive treatment on stroke recurrence. *JAMA* 1974; 229:409-418.

4. Marshall J: A trial of long-term hypotensive therapy in cerebrovascular disease. *Lancet* 1964;1:10-12.

5. Veterans Administration Cooperative Study Group on Antihypertensive Agents: Effects of treatment on morbidity in hypertension. Results in patients with diastolic blood pressures averaging 115 through 129 mm Hg. *JAMA* 1967;202:1028-1034.

6. Veterans Administration Cooperative Study Group on Antihypertensive Agents: Effects of treatment on morbidity in hypertension. II. Results in patients with diastolic blood pressure averaging 90 through 114 mm Hg. *JAMA* 1970;213:1143-1152.

7. Reynolds E, Baron RB: Hypertension in women and the elderly. Some puzzling and some expected findings of treatment studies. *Postgrad Med* 1996;100:58-63,67-70.

8. Gueyffier F, Boutitie F, Boissel JP, et al: Effect of antihypertensive drug treatment on cardiovascular outcomes in women and men. A meta-analysis of individual patient data from randomized, controlled trials. The INDANA Investigators. *Ann Intern Med* 1997;126:761-767.

9. SHEP Cooperative Research Group: Prevention of stroke by antihypertensive drug treatment in older persons with isolated systolic hypertension. Final results of the Systolic Hypertension in the Elderly Program (SHEP). *JAMA* 1991;265:3255-3264.

10. Staessen JA, Fagard R, Thijs L, et al: Randomised double-blind comparison of placebo and active treatment for older patients with isolated systolic hypertension. The Systolic Hypertension in Europe (Syst-Eur) Trial Investigators. *Lancet* 1997;350:757-764.

11. Cutler JA: Calcium-channel blockers for hypertension—uncertainty continues. *N Engl J Med* 1998;338:679-681.

12. Borhani NO, Mercuri M, Borhani PA, et al: Final outcome results of the Multicenter Isradipine Diuretic Atherosclerosis Study (MIDAS). A randomized controlled trial. *JAMA* 1996;276:785-791.

13. Furberg CD, Psaty BM, Meyer JV: Nifedipine. Dose-related increase in mortality in patients with coronary heart disease. *Circulation* 1995;92:1326-1331.

14. Estacio RO, Jeffers BW, Hiatt WR, et al: The effect of nisoldipine as compared with enalapril on cardiovascular outcomes in patients with non-insulin-dependent diabetes and hypertension. *N Engl J Med* 1998;338:645-652.

15. Davis BR, Cutler JA, Gordon DJ, et al: Rationale and design for the Antihypertensive and Lipid Lowering Treatment to Prevent Heart Attack Trial (ALLHAT). *Am J Hypertens* 1996; 9:342-360.

16. Kannel WB, McGee DL: Diabetes and cardiovascular disease. The Framingham Study. *JAMA* 1979;241:2035-2038.

17. Beach KW, Strandness DE Jr: Arteriosclerosis obliterans and associated risk factors in insulin-dependent and non-insulin-dependent diabetes. *Diabetes* 1980;29:882-888.

18. Alex M, Baron EK, Goldenberg S, et al: An autopsy study of cerebrovascular accident in diabetes mellitus. *Circulation* 1962; 25:663-673.

19. Mayne EE, Bridges JM, Weaver JA: Platelet adhesiveness, plasma fibrinogen and factor 8 levels in diabetes mellitus. *Diabetologia* 1970;6:436-440.

20. Ginsberg MD, Welsh FA, Budd WW: Deleterious effect of glucose pretreatment on recovery from diffuse cerebral ischemia in the cat. I. Local cerebral blood flow and glucose utilization. *Stroke* 1980;11:347-354.

21. Welsh FA, Ginsberg MD, Rieder W, et al: Deleterious effect of glucose pretreatment on recovery from diffuse cerebral ischemia in the cat. II. Regional metabolite levels. *Stroke* 1980; 11:355-363.

22. Weinberger J, Biscarra V, Weisberg MK, et al: Factors contributing to stroke in patients with atherosclerotic disease of the great vessels: the role of diabetes. *Stroke* 1983;14:709-712.

23. Merimee TJ: Diabetic retinopathy. A synthesis of perspectives. *N Engl J Med* 1990;322:978-983.

24. Tuomilehto J, Rastenyte D, Jousilahti P, et al: Diabetes mellitus as a risk factor for death from stroke. Prospective study of the middle-aged Finnish population. *Stroke* 1996;27:210-215.

25. Kannel WB, Wolf PA: Epidemiology of cerebrovascular disease. In: Ross-Russell RW, ed. *Vascular Disease of the Central Nervous System*, 2nd ed. New York, Churchill Livingstone, 1983, pp 1-24.

26. Konishi M, Iso H, Komachi Y, et al: Associations of serum total cholesterol, different types of stroke, and stenosis distribution of cerebral arteries. The Akita Pathology Study. *Stroke* 1993; 24:954-964.

27. Gillman MW, Cupples LA, Millen BE, et al: Inverse association of dietary fat with development of ischemic stroke in men. *JAMA* 1997;278:2145-2150.

28. Gillum RF, Mussolino ME, Madans JH: The relationship between fish consumption and stroke incidence. The NHANES I Epidemiologic Follow-up Study (National Health and Nutrition Examination Survey). *Arch Intern Med* 1996;156:537-542.

29. Gey KF, Stahelin HB, Eichholzer M: Poor plasma status of carotene and vitamin C is associated with higher mortality from ischemic heart disease and stroke: Basel Prospective Study. *Clin Investig* 1993;71:3-6.

30. Kushi LH, Folsom AR, Prineas RJ, et al: Dietary antioxidant vitamins and death from coronary heart disease in postmenopausal women. *N Engl J Med* 1996;334:1156-1162.

31. Welch GN, Loscalzo J: Homocysteine and atherothrombosis. *N Engl J Med* 1998;338:1042-1050.

32. Hebert PR, Gaziano JM, Chan KS, et al: Cholesterol lowering with statin drugs, risk of stroke, and total mortality. An overview of randomized trials. *JAMA* 1997;278:313-321.

33. Jukema JW, Bruschke AV, van Boven AJ, et al: Effects of lipid lowering by pravastatin on progression and regression of coronary artery disease in symptomatic men with normal to mod-

erately elevated serum cholesterol levels. The Regression Growth Evaluation Statin Study (REGRESS). *Circulation* 1995;91:2528-2540.

34.   The Multicentre Anti-Atheroma Study: Effect of simvastatin on coronary atheroma. *Lancet* 1994;344:633-638.

35.   The Scandinavian Simvastatin Survival Study (4S): Randomised trial of cholesterol lowering in 4444 patients with coronary heart disease. *Lancet* 1994;344:1383-1389.

36.   Shepherd J, Cobbe SM, Ford I, et al: Prevention of coronary heart disease with pravastatin in men with hypercholesterolemia. West of Scotland Coronary Prevention Study Group. *N Engl J Med* 1995;333:1301-1307.

37.   Sacks FM, Pfeffer MA, Moye LA, et al: The effect of pravastatin on coronary events after myocardial infarction in patients with average cholesterol levels. *N Engl J Med* 1996;335:1001-1009.

38.   The Long-Term Intervention with Pravastatin in Ischaemic Disease (LIPID) Study Group: Prevention of cardiovascular events and death with pravastatin in patients with coronary heart disease and a broad range of initial cholesterol levels. *N Engl J Med* 1998;339(19):1349-1357.

39.   Plehn JF, Davis BR, Sacks FM, et al: Reduction of stroke incidence after myocardial infarction with pravastatin: The Cholesterol and Recurrent Events (CARE) study. The CARE Investigators. *Circulation* 1999;99(2):216-223.

40.   Crouse JR 3d, Byington RP, Bond MG, et al: Pravastatin, Lipids, and Atherosclerosis in the Carotid Arteries (PLAC-II). *Am J Cardiol* 1995;75:455-459.

41.   Furberg CD, Adams HP Jr, Applegate WB, et al: Effect of lovastatin on early carotid atherosclerosis and cardiovascular events. Asymptomatic Carotid Artery Progression Study (ACAPS) Research Group. *Circulation* 1994;90:1679-1687.

42.   Dewarrat A, Bogousslavsky J: Antithrombotic agents and prevention of cerebrovascular accidents. *Rev Med Suisse Romande* 1996;116:629-634.

43.   Steering Committee of the Physicians' Health Study Research Group: Final report on the aspirin component of the ongoing Physicians' Health Study. *N Engl J Med* 1989;321:129-135.

44.   ISIS-2 (Second International Study of Infarct Survival) Collaborative Group: Randomised trial of intravenous streptokinase, oral aspirin, both, or neither among 17,187 cases of suspected myocardial infarction: ISIS-2. *Lancet* 1988;2:349-360.

45.   CAPRIE Steering Committee: A randomised, blinded, trial of clopidogrel versus aspirin in patients at risk of ischaemic events (CAPRIE). *Lancet* 1996;348:1329-1339.

46.   Salonen JT, Salonen R: Ultrasound B-mode imaging in observational studies of atherosclerotic progression. *Circulation* 1993;87:II56-II65.

47.   Tell GS, Howard G, McKinney WM, et al: Cigarette smoking cessation and extracranial carotid atherosclerosis. *JAMA* 1989; 261:1178-1180.

48.   Leys D, Lamy C, Lucas C, et al: Arterial ischemic strokes associated with pregnancy and puerperium. *Acta Neurol Belg* 1997;97:5-16.

49.   Kittner SJ, Stern BJ, Feeser BR, et al: Pregnancy and the risk of stroke. *N Engl J Med* 1996;335:768-774.

50.   WHO Collaborative Study of Cardiovascular Disease and Steroid Hormone Contraception: Ischaemic stroke and combined oral contraceptives: results of an international, multicentre, case-control study. *Lancet* 1996;348:498-505.

51.   Jonas HA, Kronmal RA, Psaty BM, et al: Current estrogen-progestin and estrogen replacement therapy in elderly women: association with carotid atherosclerosis. CHS Collaborative Research Group. Cardiovascular Health Study. *Ann Epidemiol* 1996;6:314-323.

52.   Sandok BA, Whisnant JP, Furlan AJ, et al: Carotid artery bruits: prevalence survey and differential diagnosis. *Mayo Clin Proc* 1982;57:227-230.

53.   Blackshear WM, Phillips DJ, Chikos PM, et al: Carotid artery velocity patterns in normal and stenotic vessels. *Stroke* 1980; 11:67-71.

54.   Suwanwela N, Can U, Furie KL, et al: Carotid Doppler ultrasound criteria for internal carotid artery stenosis based on residual lumen diameter calculated from en bloc carotid endarterectomy specimens. *Stroke* 1996;27:1965-1969.

College of the Ouachitas

55. Executive Committee for the Asymptomatic Carotid Atherosclerosis Study: Endarterectomy for asymptomatic carotid artery stenosis. *JAMA* 1995;273:1421-1428.

56. Norris JW, Zhu CZ, Bornstein NM, et al: Vascular risks of asymptomatic carotid stenosis. *Stroke* 1991;22:1485-1490.

57. Weinberger J, Ramos L, Ambrose JA, et al: Morphologic and dynamic changes of atherosclerotic plaque at the carotid artery bifurcation: sequential imaging by real time B-mode ultrasonography. *J Am Coll Cardiol* 1988;12:1515-1521.

58. Reilly LM, Lusby RJ, Hughes L, et al: Carotid plaque histology using real-time ultrasonography. Clinical and therapeutic implications. *Am J Surg* 1983;146:188-193.

59. Steffen CM, Gray-Weale AC, Byrne KE, et al: Carotid artery atheroma: ultrasound appearance in symptomatic and asymptomatic vessels. *Aust N Z J Surg* 1989;59:529-534.

60. Johnson JM, Kennelly MM, Decesare D, et al: Natural history of asymptomatic carotid plaque. *Arch Surg* 1985;120:1010-1012.

61. Weinberger J, Tegeler CH, McKinney WM, et al: Ultrasonography for diagnosis and management of carotid artery atherosclerosis. A position paper of the American Society of Neuroimaging. *J Neuroimaging* 1995;5:237-243.

62. Polak JF, Bajakian RL, O'Leary DH, et al: Detection of internal carotid artery stenosis: comparison of MR angiography, color Doppler sonography, and arteriography. *Radiology* 1992;182:35-40.

63. Furlan AJ, Craciun AR: Risk of stroke during coronary artery bypass graft surgery in patients with internal carotid artery disease documented by angiography. *Stroke* 1985;16:797-799.

64. Treiman RL, Foran RF, Cohen JL, et al: Carotid bruit: a follow-up report on its significance in patients undergoing an abdominal aortic operation. *Arch Surg* 1979;114:1138-1140.

65. Gerraty RP, Gates PC, Doyle JC: Carotid stenosis and perioperative stroke risk in symptomatic and asymptomatic patients undergoing vascular or coronary surgery. *Stroke* 1993; 24:1115-1118.

66. Wolf PA, Dawber TR, Thomas HE Jr, et al: Epidemiologic assessment of chronic atrial fibrillation and risk of stroke: the Framingham Study. *Neurology* 1978;28:973-977.

67. Atrial Fibrillation Investigators: Risk factors for stroke and efficacy of antithrombotic therapy in atrial fibrillation. Analysis of pooled data from five randomized controlled trials. *Arch Intern Med* 1994;154:1449-1457.

68. Stroke Prevention in Atrial Fibrillation Study: Final results. *Circulation* 1991;84:527-539.

69. Stroke Prevention in Atrial Fibrillation II Study: Warfarin versus aspirin for prevention of thromboembolism in atrial fibrillation. *Lancet* 1994;343:687-691.

70. The Stroke Prevention in Atrial Fibrillation Investigators: Predictors of thromboembolism in atrial fibrillation: I. Clinical features of patients at risk. *Ann Intern Med* 1992;116:1-5.

71. The Stroke Prevention in Atrial Fibrillation Investigators: Predictors of thromboembolism in atrial fibrillation: II. Echocardiographic features of patients at risk. *Ann Intern Med* 1992; 116:6-12.

72. Petersen P, Boysen G, Godtfredsen J, et al: Placebo-controlled, randomised trial of warfarin and aspirin for prevention of thromboembolic complications in chronic atrial fibrillation. The Copenhagen AFASAK study. *Lancet* 1989;1:175-179.

73. The Boston Area Anticoagulation Trial for Atrial Fibrillation Investigators: The effect of low-dose warfarin on the risk of stroke in patients with nonrheumatic atrial fibrillation. *N Engl J Med* 1990;323:1505-1511.

74. Ezekowitz MD, Bridgers SL, James KE, et al: Warfarin in the prevention of stroke associated with nonrheumatic atrial fibrillation. Veterans Affairs Stroke Prevention in Nonrheumatic Atrial Fibrillation Investigators. *N Engl J Med* 1992;327:1406-1412.

75. Szekely P: Systemic embolism and anticoagulant prophylaxis in rheumatic heart disease. *Br Med J* 1964;1:1209-1212.

76. Smith P, Arnesen H, Holme I: The effect of warfarin on mortality and reinfarction after myocardial infarction. *N Engl J Med* 1990;323:147-152.

Chapter **4**

Diagnosis and Management of Transient Ischemic Attacks

Transient ischemic attacks (TIAs) are defined as episodes of transient focal neurologic dysfunction caused by a temporary lack of blood supply to a region of the brain. Typical symptoms of a cerebral TIA are a temporary inability to speak, weakness on one side of the body, and transient sensory disturbance. Patients with vertebrobasilar insufficiency may have symptoms of focal brain stem dysfunction such as double vision or vertigo, which often are difficult to distinguish from other causes of dizziness. Transient visual loss in one eye, or amaurosis fugax, is an indication of ipsilateral carotid artery atherosclerotic disease,[1] and is clinically equivalent to a TIA.

Recognition of TIA is critical because it is a highly significant warning sign of impending stroke. Between 25% and 33% of patients with TIA develop completed stroke, most commonly within the first 3 months after the initial transient event.[2] Atherosclerotic disease at the carotid artery bifurcation is responsible for 50% of cerebral TIAs, while the other potential sources of cerebral ischemia, including cardioembolic causes and intracranial small-vessel disease, account for the remaining events.

Diagnosis of TIA

Appropriate management of TIA requires that the nature and etiology of the TIA be accurately diagnosed. The management of TIA patients is summarized in Figure 1. A frank transient hemiparesis clearly indicates that a contralateral cerebral ischemic event has occurred. When a patient develops a transient disturbance of eye movements with diplopia and a contralateral hemiparesis, a brain stem ischemic event clearly has occurred. However, many patients present with symptoms of generalized cerebral ischemia, such as syncope or lightheadedness, which may be caused by decreased brain perfusion caused by cardiac or autonomic dysfunction. These do not carry the same prognosis for focal stroke as an actual TIA. On the other hand, up to 20% of patients with these nonspecific symptoms, particularly older patients, have hemodynamically significant carotid artery occlusive disease.[3] Patients with transient visual disturbance that is not typical of amaurosis fugax have a much lower incidence of carotid artery atherosclerotic disease than do patients describing a true altitudinal shadow over the eye. However, carotid artery or vertebrobasilar occlusive disease must also be ruled out in these patients.[4] Another symptom that may be related to TIA, primarily in the vertebrobasilar circulation, is transient global amnesia, in which the patient loses memory for several hours, although other functions remain normal.[5] Occlusive vascular disease has not been associated with transient global amnesia, but is usually ruled out with noninvasive vascular studies.[6] A careful history must be taken, because some patients with structural brain lesions may have transient focal events attributable to seizure activity rather than ischemia. An imaging study of the brain is indicated in circumstances where the history suggests another cause for the transient neurologic disturbance.

Evaluation of the cerebral vasculature with ultrasonography is an accurate and convenient noninvasive method

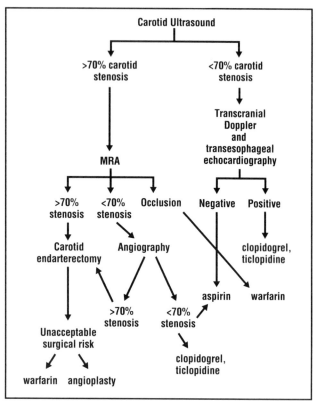

Figure 1: Diagnosis of TIA or amaurosis fugax. The flowchart describes the diagnosis and management of TIA.

for determining the extent of occlusive disease of the extracranial carotid artery bifurcation, the extracranial vertebral arteries, and both the anterior and posterior cerebral circulation.[7] Duplex Doppler color flow ultrasonography can identify a stenosis of greater than 70% with an accuracy of 90%, compared with angiography, in a laboratory that has calibrated the peak systolic velocity and end-diastolic velocity of the Doppler spectral analysis with angiographic determination of percent stenosis.[8] The Doppler frequency shift depends on the residual area of the lumen of the artery, and thus in some ways more accurately represents the degree of stenosis in pathologic specimens than does angiography, with 96% sensitivity and 61% specificity for detecting a critical residual lumen diameter of less than 1.5 mm.[9]

Doppler frequency shifts may be falsely elevated in patients with TIA because of mitral valve prolapse, but this can be distinguished by analysis of the Doppler waveform, and appropriate diagnosis can be made.[10]

Distal perfusion can be assessed by transcranial Doppler to corroborate whether an internal carotid stenosis is hemodynamically significant.[11] Hemodynamically significant lesions with residual lumen diameter less than 1.5 mm cause reversal of flow in the ophthalmic arteries or cross-filling from the contralateral carotid through the anterior communicating artery with reversal of flow in the anterior cerebral artery.[11] Transcranial Doppler can detect whether a TIA is caused by stenosis of an intracranial artery rather than stenosis at the carotid artery bifurcation. Ultrasonography of the cervical vertebral artery[12] and transcranial Doppler study of the intracranial vertebrobasilar system[13] are valuable in determining whether patients with nonspecific symptoms suggestive of vertebrobasilar insufficiency indeed have occlusive disease of the vertebral or basilar arteries.

In some centers, Doppler ultrasonography is the sole determinant of whether medical or surgical management of TIA patients is preferable. In most instances, a confirmatory imaging procedure is performed when Doppler studies suggest a hemodynamically significant lesion, or if the Doppler study is technically not definitive.[7] Magnetic resonance angiography (MRA) usually is performed because it is also noninvasive. MRA also has an accuracy of about 90% for identifying a hemodynamically significant 70%

stenosis of the internal carotid artery, and the results of Doppler and MRA complement each other. The accuracy of the two studies combined provides a 95% correlation with the results of angiography.[8] However, some clinicians insist that intra-arterial contrast angiography be performed because the studies documenting the role of carotid endarterectomy in the management of TIA are based on criteria developed with intra-arterial contrast angiography.[14]

Management of Carotid Artery TIA

Even though nonobstructive ulcerated plaques at the carotid artery bifurcation can cause symptoms of TIA and stroke,[15,16] researchers have known for several years that patients with greater than 70% hemodynamically significant carotid artery stenosis are at greater risk for stroke.[17] However, in the past, whether patients with carotid artery stenosis and TIA benefited more from medical therapy or surgical intervention was not clear, because the risk of stroke or adverse outcome with carotid endarterectomy was almost as great as the risk of stroke with no treatment.[18] More recently, patients with carotid artery TIA or amaurosis fugax had significantly better results with surgery than with medical therapy (aspirin 650 mg b.i.d.) when stenosis of the origin of the ipsilateral internal carotid artery was greater than 70%[14] (Figure 2). The risk of stroke ipsilateral to a 70% carotid artery stenosis was 2% with surgical management and 20% with medical management.[14] Selected patients with 50% to 70% stenosis also benefit from carotid endarterectomy, specifically nondiabetic men.[19] Accurate quantification of the degree of carotid stenosis in TIA patients has become imperative, and patients with the appropriate degree of stenosis are referred for carotid endarterectomy unless they have overwhelming medical contraindications to surgery. In these cases, angioplasty and stenting of the internal carotid artery may be valuable, but the number of complications with stenting is equal to the number with carotid endart-

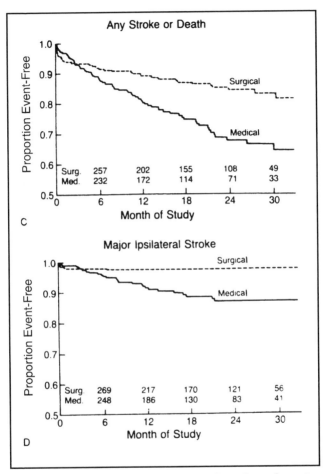

Figure 2: The results of the North American Symptomatic Carotid Endarterectomy Trial. There is a significant reduction in any stroke or death and in major stroke ipsilateral to the stenotic carotid artery with carotid endarterectomy, compared with medical therapy with aspirin 650 mg twice a day when carotid stenosis is greater than 70%.[14] Used with permission.

erectomy in controlled studies, and the long-term outcome of stenting has not been established.[20]

Surgical therapy for carotid endarterectomy, when indicated, must be performed in a considerably experienced center. The incidence of stroke complications in the major centers involved in the controlled trials of carotid endarterectomy was less than 2%, and the 30-day mortality was extremely low: 0.6% in NASCET and 0.1% in ACAS.[21] A review of Medicare recipients undergoing carotid endarterectomy in 1992 and 1993 revealed a perioperative mortality rate of 1.4% in hospitals involved in clinical trials.[21] In nontrial hospitals, the mortality rate was directly related to the volume of operations performed, with a rate of 1.7% in high-volume centers, 1.9% in average-volume centers, and 2.3% in low-volume centers.[21] Because of the higher risk of surgery in the community than the risk reported in clinical trials, the clinician must also be certain that a patient has actually had a TIA directly related to a carotid artery stenosis rather than a nonspecific symptom such as dizziness, in which case the patient should be treated like a patient with asymptomatic carotid stenosis.[22]

Medical Therapy of TIA

Medical therapy for patients with TIA is indicated for patients with nonsurgical lesions of the carotid artery, patients with cerebral TIA without carotid artery stenosis, patients with intracranial vascular disease not amenable to surgical treatment, and patients with vertebrobasilar circulation TIA. The standard medical treatment for patients with TIA is the platelet antiaggregant aspirin, although in most studies the etiology of the TIA was not taken into account. Aspirin inhibits the enzyme cyclooxygenase, which produces the prostaglandin thromboxane from arachidonic acid.[23] Thromboxane is a strong inducer of platelet aggregation in vitro.

Aspirin

The Canadian Cooperative Study was the first large, multicenter, controlled trial of aspirin in patients with TIA. Aspirin 650 mg by mouth twice a day significantly reduced the incidence of subsequent stroke by 50% in men, although no statistically significant reduction was found in women.[24] Subsequent trials used lower dosages of aspirin based on the hypothesis that a high dose of aspirin also inhibited prostacyclin, another prostaglandin formed by cyclooxygenase that is present in arterial walls and prevents thrombosis.[25] Several studies showed a significant reduction of stroke in patients with TIA treated with low dosages of aspirin, from 30 to 283 mg/d.[26-28] However, a comparison of studies using doses of aspirin <975 mg/d and those with doses of >975 mg/d showed a significantly greater reduction in stroke in the higher-dosage group.[29] Meta-analysis of these aspirin studies also showed a significant beneficial effect of aspirin therapy in preventing stroke in women with symptomatic TIA.[29,30] Therefore, a dosage of aspirin of 975 mg/d is recommended in patients with TIA, or the highest tolerable dosage of aspirin up to 975 mg/d if the patient has difficulty tolerating the high dose because of gastrointestinal discomfort. Several agents can reduce the gastrointestinal discomfort or bleeding associated with aspirin, including misoprostol (Cytotec®) 1,000 mg q.i.d., the histamine$_2$-receptor antagonists such as ranitidine (Zantac®), cimetidine (Tagamet®), and famotidine (Pepcid®), or the proton-pump inhibitor omeprazole (Prilosec®). These agents can make the high dose of aspirin more tolerable.

Ticlopidine

Another platelet antiaggregant drug, ticlopidine (Ticlid®), was developed for patients with TIA who could not tolerate aspirin and for women, because of the possibility that aspirin was not as effective in women as in men. Ticlopidine prevents platelet aggregation by blocking the

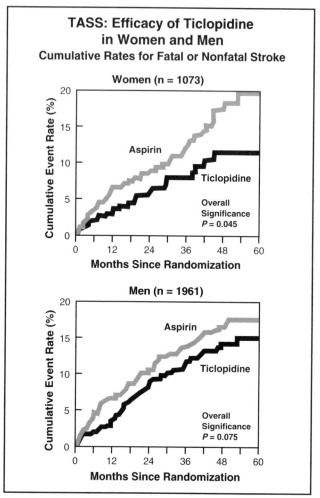

Figure 3: *The results of the Ticlopidine Aspirin Stroke Study (TASS) showing a greater effect of ticlopidine in preventing stroke in both male and female TIA patients compared with aspirin, with an even greater effect in women than in men.[32] Used with permission.*

adenosine diphosphate receptor.[31] Ticlopidine prevents in vitro platelet aggregation to a broader spectrum of stimuli than aspirin, and further prolongs bleeding time.[32]

In a study of patients with focal TIA and amaurosis fugax, ticlopidine was found to be more effective than aspirin 650 mg by mouth twice a day in preventing stroke, with a relative risk reduction of 48% after 1 year of treatment and 25% after 5 years of treatment[32] (Figure 3). In this study, different etiologies of TIA were analyzed. Ticlopidine appeared to be as equally effective as aspirin in preventing stroke from carotid artery disease, but was more effective than aspirin in patients with intracranial vascular disease.[32] Ticlopidine had a beneficial effect over aspirin in female patients[32] and in African-American patients.[33]

Patients taking ticlopidine must be monitored for complications. The risk of clinically significant neutropenia is 2%, as well as a lesser degree of thrombocytopenia and hepatic toxicity.[32] Most adverse events occur within the first 3 months of therapy, and are reversible if the drug is discontinued. However, there have been two reports of irreversible neutropenia, and a warning has been issued that ticlopidine can cause acute thrombotic thrombocytopenic purpura (TTP). The white blood count, platelet count, and liver function tests must be monitored every 2 weeks for the first 3 months of treatment so the medication can be discontinued if toxicity occurs. Because of its associated adverse events, ticlopidine is generally used when a TIA patient cannot tolerate aspirin, or when TIA recurs despite aspirin therapy. Ticlopidine is sometimes used as the primary antiplatelet agent for TIA in women, in patients with intracranial vascular disease, and in African-American patients.

Clopidogrel

Clopidogrel (Plavix®) is a new platelet antiaggregant agent that acts by direct inhibition of adenosine diphosphate (ADP), binding to its receptor, and of the subsequent ADP-mediated activation of the GPIIB/IIIA complex. Clopidogrel is not associated with the severe hematologic adverse events of ticlopidine, including neutropenia, thrombocytopenia, and TTP. Therefore, routine hematologic monitoring is not required with clopidogrel. Clopidogrel has a lower incidence of gastrointestinal disturbances that occur with aspirin, including indigestion, nausea, and vomiting, as well as gastrointestinal hemorrhage.[34] Clopidogrel was compared to aspirin for prevention of ischemic events in patients with atherosclerotic vascular disease in the CAPRIE Study.[34] Patients with recent ischemic stroke, recent myocardial infarction, or established peripheral arterial disease were treated with either aspirin 325 mg/d or clopidogrel 75 mg/d. A statistically significant 8.7% relative risk reduction occurred in subsequent events of ischemic stroke, myocardial infarction, or vascular death among patients taking clopidogrel, compared with the patients taking aspirin.[34] Clopidogrel has not been directly compared to aspirin in a study to determine whether it is more effective for preventing stroke in patients with TIA, and has not been directly compared to ticlopidine to determine if it is equally effective. However, in all patients in the CAPRIE trial with a history of cerebrovascular disease (TIA, reversible ischemic neurologic deficit, amaurosis fugax, and stroke), there was an 8.3% risk reduction compared with aspirin for the combined outcome of stroke, MI, and vascular death.[35] This benefit of clopidogrel over aspirin occurred in both lacunar and nonlacunar stroke.[36] Therefore, clopidogrel is a good choice for treatment of patients with TIA who cannot tolerate aspirin therapy, or in treating patients who have cerebral ischemic events while on aspirin therapy, and possibly as primary therapy in the subcategories of patients with TIA.

Dipyridamole

Dipyridamole (Persantine®) prevents platelet aggregation by inhibiting the enzyme phosphodiesterase.[37] Inhibition of this enzyme may also have vasodilatory effects. Initial studies showed that dipyridamole was not effective in preventing strokes in patients with TIA when administered alone,[37] and did not have an additive effect in preventing strokes when administered with aspirin,[38] when compared to aspirin alone. These negative results may be partly attributable to the higher doses of aspirin used in the trials or to the side effects of headache and dizziness that occurred with the multiple dosing regimens of dipyridamole, which may have reduced patient compliance.

A more recent trial, the Second European Stroke Prevention Study, used a time-release preparation of dipyridamole 400 mg/d. This dosage was equivalent to low-dose aspirin 50 mg/d in reducing the relative risk of stroke by 18%.[39] The combination of time-release dipyridamole 400 mg/d with aspirin 50 mg/d resulted in a 37% risk reduction of stroke when compared to placebo.[39] This very low dose of aspirin and very high dose of dipyridamole may have biased the study in favor of dipyridamole since earlier studies showed no additional benefit of adding dipyridamole to high-dose aspirin. The combination of low-dose aspirin and time-release dipyridamole (Aggrenox®) appears equivalent to high-dose aspirin in prevention of stroke; however, the combination did not reduce the risk of myocardial infarction when compared to aspirin alone. This combination can be used by TIA patients who cannot tolerate the gastrointestinal effects of high-dose aspirin or the dizziness associated with the standard preparation of dipyridamole.

Warfarin

Warfarin (Coumadin®) is used as initial therapy for prevention of stroke in patients with a cardiogenic source of emboli who have had a TIA. Patients with atrial fibrillation may have a TIA as their first manifestation of cerebrovascular disease. These patients require anticoagulation with warfarin. Echocardiography is generally performed for TIA patients without an atherosclerotic or hypertensive etiology. Patients with mitral valve prolapse may present with TIA. While aspirin is effective in preventing stroke in most patients with mitral valve prolapse,[40] patients with large redundant valves with myxomatous changes may require warfarin for stroke prophylaxis. TIA patients with ventricular wall abnormalities or dilated cardiomyopathy also should be treated with warfarin.

Transesophageal echocardiography should be performed in patients with no clear source of TIA to identify occult sources such as aortic arch plaque,[41] patent foramen ovale,[42] or atrial septal aneurysm. Prophylactic therapy with warfarin to prevent stroke is indicated in TIA patients with patent foramen ovale or atrial abnormalities,[42] and was recently shown to be effective in patients with aortic arch plaque with mobile thrombus.[43]

Warfarin is more effective than aspirin in preventing recurrence in stroke patients with large-vessel intracranial vascular occlusive disease.[44] Therefore, warfarin is commonly used in TIA patients with large-vessel occlusive disease whose condition is not controlled with aspirin, and is often used as primary therapy in patients with vertebrobasilar TIA from large-vessel occlusive disease.

Conclusion

Both medical and surgical therapy exist for prevention of stroke in patients with TIA. As with completed stroke, the etiology of the TIA must be defined to prescribe adequate prophylactic therapy. The indications for carotid artery endarterectomy have become more clearly defined, and new medical treatments that are more effective than aspirin have been developed. Carotid artery stenting may become standard therapy in the treatment of carotid artery disease, but its efficacy has not been established.

References

1.   Fisher CM: Transient monocular blindness associated with hemiplegia. *Arch Ophthalmol* 1952;47:167-203.

2.   Mohr JP: Transient ischemic attacks and the prevention of strokes. *N Engl J Med* 1978;299:93-95.

3.   Weinberger J, Biscarra V, Weisberg MK: Hemodynamics of the carotid-artery circulation in the elderly "dizzy" patient. *J Am Geriatr Soc* 1981;29:402-406.

4.   Gaul JJ, Marks SJ, Weinberger J: Visual disturbance and carotid artery disease. 500 symptomatic patients studied by non-invasive carotid artery testing including B-mode ultrasonography. *Stroke* 1986;17:393-398.

5.   Bender MB: Syndrome of isolated episode of confusion with amnesia. *J Hillside Hosp* 1956;5:212-215.

6.   Feuer D, Weinberger J: Extracranial carotid artery in patients with transient global amnesia: evaluation by real-time B-mode ultrasonography with duplex Doppler flow. *Stroke* 1987;18:951-953.

7.   Weinberger J, Tegeler CH, McKinney WM, et al: Ultrasonography for diagnosis and management of carotid artery atherosclerosis. A position paper of the American Society of Neuroimaging. *J Neuroimaging* 1995;5:237-243.

8.   Polak JF, Bajakian RL, O'Leary DH, et al: Detection of internal carotid artery stenosis: comparison of MR angiography, color Doppler sonography, and arteriography. *Radiology* 1992;182:35-40.

9.   Suwanwela N, Can U, Furie KL, et al: Carotid Doppler ultrasound criteria for internal carotid artery stenosis based on residual lumen diameter calculated from en bloc carotid endarterectomy specimens. *Stroke* 1996;27:1965-1969.

10.   Weinberger J, Goldman M: Detection of mitral valve abnormalities by carotid Doppler flow study: implications for the management of patients with cerebrovascular disease. *Stroke* 1985; 16:977-980.

11.   Can U, Furie KL, Suwanwela N, et al: Transcranial Doppler ultrasound criteria for hemodynamically significant internal carotid artery stenosis based on residual lumen diameter calculated

from en bloc endarterectomy specimens. *Stroke* 1997;28: 1966-1971.

12. Weinberger J: Noninvasive imaging of the cervical vertebral artery in the diagnosis of vertebrobasilar insufficiency. *J Stroke Cerebrovasc Dis* 1991;1:21-25.

13. Ringelstein EB: A practical guide to transcranial Doppler sonography. In: Weinberger J, ed. *Noninvasive Imaging of Cerebrovascular Disease.* New York, Alan R. Liss, 1989, pp 75-121.

14. North American Symptomatic Carotid Endarterectomy Trial Collaborators: Beneficial effect of carotid endarterectomy in symptomatic patients with high-grade carotid stenosis. *N Engl J Med* 1991;325:445-453.

15. Moore WS, Hall AD: Importance of emboli from carotid bifurcation in pathogenesis of cerebral ischemic attacks. *Arch Surg* 1970;101:708-711.

16. Weinberger J, Robbins A: Neurologic symptoms associated with nonobstructive plaque at carotid bifurcation. Analysis by real-time B-mode ultrasonography. *Arch Neurol* 1983;40:489-492.

17. Weinberger J, Biscarra V, Weitzner I Jr, et al: Noninvasive carotid artery testing; role in management of patients with transient ischemic attacks. *N Y State J Med* 1981;81:1463-1468.

18. Fields WS, Maslenikov V, Meyer JS, et al: Joint study of extracranial arterial occlusion. V. Progress report of prognosis following surgery or nonsurgical treatment for transient cerebral ischemic attacks and cervical carotid artery lesions. *JAMA* 1970; 211:1993-2003.

19. Barnett HJ, Taylor DW, Eliasziw M: Benefit of carotid endarterectomy in patients with symptomatic moderate or severe stenosis. North American Symptomatic Carotid Endarterectomy Trial Collaborators. *N Engl J Med* 1998;339:1415-1425.

20. Diethrich EB, Ndiaye M, Reid DB: Stenting in the carotid artery: initial experience in 110 patients. *J Endovasc Surg* 1996; 3:42-62.

21. Wennberg DE, Lucas FL, Birkmeyer JD, et al: Variation in carotid endarterectomy mortality in the Medicare population: trial hospitals, volume, and patient characteristics. *JAMA* 1998; 279:1278-1281.

22. Cebul RD, Snow RJ, Pine R, et al: Indications, outcomes, and provider volumes for carotid endarterectomy. *JAMA* 1998; 279:1282-1287.

23. Roth GJ, Majerus PW: The mechanism of the effect of aspirin on human platelets. I. Acetylation of a particulate fraction protein. *J Clin Invest* 1975;56:624-632.

24. The Canadian Cooperative Study Group: A randomized trial of aspirin and sulfinpyrazone in threatened stroke. *N Engl J Med* 1978;299:53-59.

25. Spranger M, Aspey BS, Harrison MJ: Sex difference in antithrombotic effect of aspirin. *Stroke* 1989;20:34-37.

26. The Dutch TIA Trial Study Group: A comparison of two doses of aspirin (30 mg vs. 283 mg a day) in patients after a transient ischemic attack or minor ischemic stroke. *N Engl J Med* 1991; 325:1261-1266.

27. The SALT Collaborative Group: Swedish Aspirin Low-Dose Trial (SALT) of 75 mg aspirin as secondary prophylaxis after cerebrovascular ischaemic events. *Lancet* 1991;338:1345-1349.

28. Farrell B, Godwin J, Richards S, et al: The United Kingdom transient ischaemic attack (UK-TIA) aspirin trial: final results. *J Neurol Neurosurg Psychiatry* 1991;54:1044-1054.

29. Dyken ML, Barnett HJ, Easton JD, et al: Low-dose aspirin and stroke. "It ain't necessarily so". *Stroke* 1992;23:1395-1399.

30. Antiplatelet Trialists' Collaboration: Secondary prevention of vascular disease by prolonged antiplatelet treatment. *Br Med J (Clin Res Ed)* 1988;296:320-331.

31. Hardisty RM, Powling MJ, Nokes TJ: The action of ticlopidine on human platelets. Studies on aggregation, secretion, calcium mobilization and membrane glycoproteins. *Thromb Haemost* 1990;64:150-155.

32. Hass WK, Easton JD, Adams HP Jr, et al: A randomized trial comparing ticlopidine hydrochloride with aspirin for the prevention of stroke in high-risk patients. Ticlopidine Aspirin Stroke Study Group. *N Engl J Med* 1989;321:501-507.

33. Grotta JC, Norris JW, Kamm B: Prevention of stroke with ticlopidine: who benefits most? TASS Baseline and Angiographic Data Subgroup. *Neurology* 1992;42:111-115.

34. CAPRIE Steering Committee: A randomised, blinded trial of clopidogrel versus aspirin in patients at risk of ischaemic events (CAPRIE). *Lancet* 1996;348:1329-1339.

35. Easton JD: Benefit of clopidogrel in patients with evidence of cerebrovascular disease. *Neurology* 1998;51:332.

36. Hacke W: Consistency of the benefit of clopidogrel over aspirin in patients with lacunar and non-lacunar stroke. The CAPRIE Investigators. *Cerebrovasc Dis* 1998;8:51.

37. Acheson J, Danta G, Hutchinson EC: Controlled trial of dipyridamole in cerebral vascular disease. *Br Med J* 1969;1:614-615.

38. The American-Canadian Co-Operative Study Group: Persantine Aspirin Trial in cerebral ischemia. Part II: Endpoint results. *Stroke* 1985;16:406-415.

39. European Stroke Prevention Study 2: Efficacy and safety data. *J Neurol Sci* 1997;151:S1-S77.

40. Barnett HJ, Boughner DR, Taylor DW, et al: Further evidence relating mitral-valve prolapse to cerebral ischemic events. *N Engl J Med* 1980;302:139-144.

41. Tunick PA, Culliford AT, Lamparello PJ, et al: Atheromatosis of the aortic arch as an occult source of multiple systemic emboli. *Ann Intern Med* 1991;114:391-392.

42. Jeanrenaud X, Kappenberger L: Patent foramen ovale and stroke of unknown origin. *Cerebrovasc Dis* 1991;1:184-192.

43. Dressler FA, Craig WR, Castello R, et al: Mobile aortic atheroma and systemic emboli: efficacy of anticoagulation and influence of plaque morphology on recurrent stroke. *J Am Coll Cardiol* 1998;31:134-138.

44. Chimowitz MI, Kokkinos J, Strong J, et al: The Warfarin-Aspirin Symptomatic Intracranial Disease Study. *Neurology* 1995;45:1488-1493.

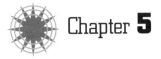 Chapter **5**

Management of Acute Ischemic Stroke: The Brain Attack

The management of acute ischemic stroke has dramatically evolved over the last decade. One treatment can actually reverse the symptoms and signs of stroke: thrombolytic therapy with tissue plasminogen activator (tPA) (recombinant alteplase, Activase®). tPA is only effective in the first 3 hours after onset of acute ischemic stroke; however, most patients do not reach the hospital within this therapeutic time window. Nevertheless, the understanding of the pathophysiology of ischemic stroke and the concept of individualizing therapy based on the type of stroke have contributed to improved treatment for all stroke patients.

Treatment of acute stroke should accomplish four main objectives: (1) treatment of associated medical conditions that could be life-threatening or worsen the ischemic deficit; (2) prevention of progression of the initial stroke; (3) prevention of recurrent stroke; and (4) reversal of the symptoms of the current stroke.

Treatment of Associated Medical Conditions

The acute presentation of stroke patients can vary considerably, ranging from an alert patient with a mild focal neurologic deficit to a patient who is severely obtunded or comatose. Immediate attention must be directed at the basic vital functions: airway patency, pulse, and blood pressure, particularly if the patient is unresponsive. Patients with ischemic stroke rarely require endotracheal intubation, but the airway should be protected from secretions to prevent aspiration. Frequent suctioning, positioning of the patient, and not feeding a patient with difficulty swallowing usually suffice.

Myocardial infarction and stroke occur concomitantly in about 10% of patients, although whether the myocardial infarction precipitates stroke or stroke provokes myocardial infarction is unclear.[1] Myocardial infarction can induce stroke by decreased perfusion or thrombotic emboli from an akinetic ventricular wall. Thromboembolic phenomena usually occur about 48 hours after the initial myocardial infarction.[2] Stroke may cause myocardial infarction through increased release of catecholamines.[3] A hypercoagulable state with increased fibrinogen production can occur after either stroke or myocardial infarction, which can cause thrombosis of coronary vessels or cerebral vessels.[4]

Abnormalities in the electrocardiogram (EKG) that can resemble the changes of myocardial infarction, including ST segment depressions and U waves, can occur in large acute strokes. Ventricular arrhythmias, including fibrillation and torsades de pointes, can occur, probably secondary to endocardial damage from catecholamine release.[5,6] Patients with stroke may also be in atrial fibrillation, and dangerously rapid atrial fibrillation can occur in association with acute stroke.

An EKG should be immediately performed in stroke patients, and serial serum myocardial enzyme analysis should be performed in suspicious cases. Ideally, stroke patients are initially hospitalized in acute stroke units with monitored beds to observe for associated cardiac arrhythmias and changes of acute myocardial infarction.[7]

Blood pressure often is elevated for about 48 hours after the onset of acute stroke, even in patients without a history of hypertension. This elevation of blood pressure usually resolves without treatment,[8] and probably is beneficial in the initial stages of stroke by maintaining perfusion of the ischemic zone around the area of infarction that is still viable, the ischemic penumbra.[9] If the blood pressure rises above a critical level, such as 200/120, moderate reduction in blood pressure with intravenous labetalol (Trandate®, Normodyne®) or oral (but not sublingual) calcium channel blockers, such as nifedipine (Adalat®, Procardia®) are used to lower the pressure to the 180/100 range. Drastic reduction in blood pressure with agents such as nitroprusside can cause deterioration of the stroke, and should be avoided.

Serum glucose may be elevated in acute ischemic stroke, even in nondiabetic patients.[10] In animal models of stroke, hyperglycemia increased the amount of ischemic damage,[11,12] and may contribute to the extent of infarction in stroke patients.[13] However, dramatically reducing blood sugar may jeopardize the ischemic penumbra. Therefore, moderate control of blood sugar is recommended once ischemic infarction has occurred.[14]

Patients who are immobilized from stroke usually are treated with subcutaneous heparin, 5,000 units b.i.d., to prevent thrombophlebitis and resultant pulmonary emboli if full anticoagulation is not employed. If the risk of cerebral or systemic bleeding is substantial, pressurized air boots can be used instead of low-dose anticoagulation. Stroke patients should be carefully monitored for respiratory compromise. Observation of oxygen saturation with a pulse oximeter is valuable in the initial stages after stroke. Patients are generally not fed if any obtundation or difficulty swallowing is present, usually for 48 hours. If inability to swallow is prolonged, a nasogastric tube or percutaneous gastric tube must be inserted to maintain nutrition for better recovery.[15] Even with precaution against aspiration, bronchopneumonia develops in obtunded patients who are unable to cough and clear their secretions.[16] Neurogenic pulmonary edema also can develop in stroke patients because of systemic vasoconstriction caused by catecholamine release.[17]

Patients with large ischemic strokes can become more obtunded during the first 24 to 72 hours after onset. This is usually caused by cerebral edema, which can, rarely, even cause brain herniation and death. The edema usually subsides spontaneously with time, and treatment is not necessary. In patients with severe obtundation that could contribute to pulmonary compromise and indicate impending brain herniation, treatment with the corticosteroid dexamethasone and osmotic diuretics may be necessary. Although the general usefulness of dexamethasone treatment for stroke patients has never been established, the subset of patients with large infarction and progressive obtundation may benefit.[18,19] In cases of acute herniation, mannitol 100 g is administered intravenously while dexamethasone is being started. Intravenous administration of glycerol (50 g in 500 mL 5% dextrose) also has been shown to enhance recovery of stroke patients.[20]

Brain edema with significant mass effect occurs in about 10% of patients with infarction from middle cerebral artery occlusion.[21] As many as 80% of these patients develop transtentorial herniation and die.[21] Moderate hypothermia[22] and decompressive surgery by removing the overlying calvarium[23] have shown favorable outcomes in uncontrolled trials, but these strategies have not yet come into general use.

Seizures also can develop in about 10% of acute stroke patients.[24] Focal spike activity or periodic lateralizing epileptiform discharges (PLEDs) can be seen on electroencephalogram (EEG), indicating the possibility of recurrent seizures.[25] Seizures usually can be controlled with anticonvulsant medications, usually phenytoin (Dilantin®), which can be conveniently administered intravenously at 50 mg/minute up to 18 mg/kg for initial loading, and orally or intravenously 100 mg every 6 to 8 hours for maintenance therapy.[24,25]

Prevention of Progression of Stroke

To prevent progression of stroke, stroke patients must be carefully observed to identify new signs or symptoms related to the stroke. An acute stroke unit that has nurses trained to identify the onset of new neurologic findings is the optimal setting for monitoring acute stroke patients.

Anticoagulation

Progression of stroke can occur in both large-vessel and small-vessel occlusive disease. Immediate anticoagulation of every stroke patient with intravenous heparin has not been effective in improving outcome in controlled clinical trials.[26] Patients with large-vessel occlusive disease who show signs of evolving stroke may benefit from anticoagulation with heparin,[27,28] particularly when brain stem infarction is present.[29] However, the deterioration must be an onset of new or progressive focal neurologic signs, such as worsening of a hemiparesis or a new cranial nerve abnormality, such as an oculomotor nerve paralysis. A decline in level of consciousness without new focal deficits is more often associated with edema secondary to reperfusion. In this instance, anticoagulation can be deleterious and should not be administered because of hemorrhagic transformation of the infarction.

Anticoagulation should be judiciously used in patients more than 80 years old who have a higher risk of hemorrhagic complications. Anticoagulation usually is ineffective in preventing progression of lacunar stroke from small-vessel disease, and should be avoided in patients with labile hypertension.

Heparin is usually administered at 1,000 units/h, and the effectiveness of anticoagulation is periodically measured with the partial thromboplastin time (PTT). When high-level anticoagulation is desired, the PTT is maintained between 70 and 80 seconds. For elderly and hypertensive patients, the PTT is usually maintained between 50 and 70 seconds. Bolus infusions usually are not performed because of the risk of hemorrhage, but can be given when immediate anticoagulation is deemed necessary.

Immediate anticoagulation may be indicated in certain instances. A brain stem stroke that is likely to progress can be clinically diagnosed when a pontine infarct is rostral to the facial nucleus, with weakness of the ipsilateral face, arm, and leg.[30] This lesion involves the ventral anterior pons where the pyramidal tracts carrying motor fibers from each cerebral hemisphere are located contiguously. Spread of infarction to both sides of the pons can result in the locked-in state, where quadraparesis and inability to speak are present, but the patient remains fully conscious. This type of stroke often is associated with basilar artery occlusion. Identification and early administration of heparin for these patients may be beneficial in preventing worsening of the ischemic infarction.

A recent study of intravenous administration of the low-molecular-weight heparinoid danaparoid (Organan™) confirmed that early anticoagulation of all stroke patients does not improve outcome at 3-month follow-up compared to placebo, although a significant beneficial effect was noted at 7 days after onset.[31] Ischemic subtype analysis showed a significant beneficial effect of early anticoagulation in patients with stroke from large-vessel occlusive disease. Patients with extracranial carotid artery occlusive disease treated acutely with danaparoid had significantly better outcomes at 3 months than patients treated with placebo.[32] Therefore, examination of the extracranial carotid artery and intracranial circulation with either carotid and transcranial Doppler ultrasonography or magnetic resonance angiography should be performed promptly in stroke patients to identify large-vessel occlusive disease so these patients can be selectively anticoagulated.

Subcutaneous administration of low-molecular-weight heparin showed a significant beneficial outcome for stroke

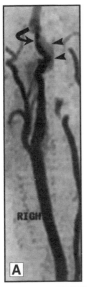

Figure 1: Magnetic resonance angiography of the internal carotid artery reveals a dissection in the wall of the artery with the true lumen (curved arrow) surrounded by thrombus from the dissection (arrowheads) in a lateral view (A) and in an axial view (B) with the surrounding thrombus indicated by the arrow. *Courtesy of Dr. Adam Silvers.*

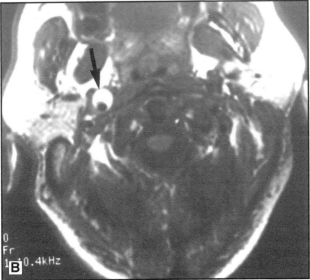

patients in one trial,[33] but was not substantiated by the International Stroke Trial.[34]

Dissection of the wall of the extracranial and intracranial internal carotid arteries and vertebral arteries also can produce an evolving stroke.[35] Dissection can occur from trauma, sometimes associated with chiropractic manipulation of the cervical spine, or spontaneously from cystic medial necrosis. Diagnosis can be made when the patient complains of neck or head pain in association with the onset of stroke. Thrombus forms between the intima and the media, compressing the lumen of the affected artery (Figure 1). When symptoms are progressive, heparin is administered to prevent complete thrombosis of the compressed true lumen, but whether all patients with dissection require anticoagulation is controversial because this might increase the amount of blood accumulating within the wall of the artery.[36] Dissection may also be a source of recurrent stroke, particularly when an open communication exists between the true and false lumen that can cause embolization of thrombus.[37] This can sometimes be identified with B-mode sonography (Figure 2), or can be deduced when multiple areas of infarction are seen on MRI (Figure 3). Anticoagulation with heparin is indicated in these instances.

Prevention of Recurrence

Anticoagulation

Prevention of recurrent stroke is essential in patients with a cardioembolic source of stroke, such as atrial fibrillation or cardiac valve replacement, to prevent further embolization from the heart.[38] Cardioembolic stroke almost always causes red infarction, with petechial hemorrhage or hemorrhagic transformation of the infarct, with regression of the embolic clot and reperfusion 24 to 48 hours after infarction.[39,40] Early anticoagulation with heparin can increase hemorrhagic transformation

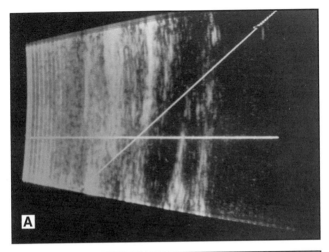

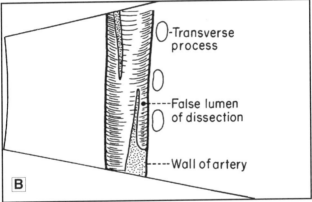

Figure 2: Real-time B-mode ultrasonogram (A) shown in schematic (B) of an angiographically documented vertebral artery dissection with an opening of the false lumen into the true lumen, serving as a source of emboli. From Weinberger J, et al: Evidence for arterial embolization in dissecting aneurysm of the cervical vertebral artery. J Stroke Cerebrovasc Dis 1991;1:95-97. Used with permission.

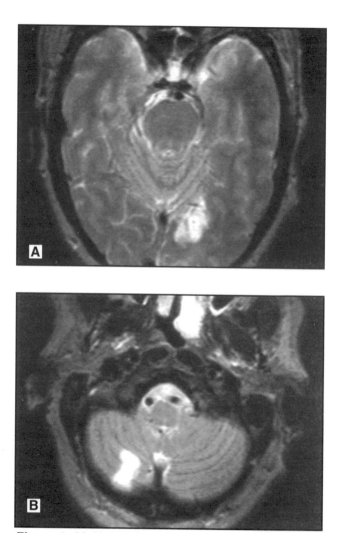

Figure 3: Multiple infarcts in the left occipital lobe (A) and right cerebellar hemisphere (B) in the same patient as in Figure 2 with T2-weighted MRI. From Weinberger J, as in Figure 2. Used with permission.

and worsen focal neurologic deficit, as well as lead to coma and death from brain herniation.

Several studies have determined that the risk of reembolization in patients with atrial fibrillation within the first 48 hours after stroke is about 2%, while the risk of major hemorrhagic transformation resulting in significant clinical deterioration is about 8%.[38-40] Anticoagulation of patients in atrial fibrillation with heparin[41] or with danaparoid[31] has shown no advantage within the first week after onset of stroke. Therefore, in patients with atrial fibrillation, anticoagulation is usually withheld for the first 48 hours, computed tomography (CT) scan of the brain is repeated, and anticoagulation is initiated if the infarct is not very large and no hemorrhagic transformation is present. In patients with large infarction involving most of the middle cerebral artery territory, or in patients with hemorrhagic transformation of the infarction, anticoagulation usually is safe 1 week after the acute onset of stroke.[42]

In patients with focal neurologic deficit, a normal initial CT scan does not indicate that anticoagulation is safe because the full extent of the lesion may not be detected until up to 48 hours after the initial event. Magnetic resonance imaging (MRI), particularly with the diffusion technique, is more sensitive in identifying the full extent of early infarction, and when the region of ischemic brain on these studies is small, anticoagulation can be instituted earlier than 48 hours.

Early anticoagulation with heparin may be necessary in patients with prosthetic cardiac valves who have a stroke while already being anticoagulated with warfarin (Coumadin®). In these patients, the risk of early reembolization is greater than the risk of anticoagulation if residual thrombus still exists on the valve. Transesophageal echocardiography should be immediately performed in these patients to identify any noninfectious vegetations suggestive of thrombus on the valve. Bacterial endocarditis must be differentiated from thrombus before anticoagulation, because mycotic aneurysms can arise from infectious emboli and cause hemorrhage when the patient is anticoagulated.[43]

Long-term anticoagulation with warfarin can be started shortly after anticoagulation is achieved with heparin to shorten the length of hospital stay. However, heparin usually is started before warfarin because, in rare instances when there is a deficiency of the vitamin K-dependent anticoagulant proteins C and S, a hypercoagulable state can occur in the early stages of warfarin therapy, which can worsen the cerebral ischemic deficit. Warfarin is usually started with a loading dose of 10 mg/d for 48 hours. Subsequent doses are titrated to the prothrombin time (PT). An international normalized ratio (INR) between 2.5 and 3.0 is optimal in most patients. In patients with prosthetic cardiac valves, an INR above 3.0 is recommended, while in elderly or high-risk patients, an INR between 2.0 and 2.5 is optimal.

Warfarin also was shown to be more effective than aspirin in prevention of recurrent stroke in patients with large-vessel intracranial vascular disease in a retrospective study.[44] This finding is being evaluated in a prospective trial, but patients who have been acutely anticoagulated with heparin because of large-vessel occlusive disease are ordinarily maintained on warfarin therapy for 3 to 6 months. Chronic maintenance warfarin therapy also usually is administered to stroke patients who test positive for anticardiolipin or antiphospholipid antibody.

Platelet Antiaggregant Therapy

Ticlopidine (Ticlid®) was the first platelet antiaggregant agent with demonstrated efficacy in preventing recurrent stroke. The Canadian American Ticlopidine Study showed a 25% risk reduction of recurrent stroke with ticlopidine 250 mg b.i.d. compared with placebo.[45] The International Stroke Trial recently demonstrated that aspirin, 300 mg/d, reduces the proportion of patients with poor outcome from stroke by 10%, primarily by preventing recurrent stroke.[30] Clopidogrel (Plavix®) also has been shown to reduce the incidence of subsequent atherosclerotic ischemic events in patients with ischemic stroke.[46]

The CAPRIE Study demonstrated that clopidogrel was 8.7% more effective than aspirin in patients with atherosclerotic disease (ischemic stroke, myocardial infarction, and peripheral arterial disease) in reducing the combined risk of ischemic stroke, myocardial infarction, and vascular death. However, the study was not designed to evaluate individual patient subgroups. In the stroke subgroup (n=6,400), there was a 7.3% risk reduction (95% CI, -5.7 to 18.7) over aspirin for the outcome of myocardial infarction, stroke, and vascular death.

Patients who do not receive anticoagulation for acute stroke should be treated with platelet antiaggregant therapy. A controlled trial is under way to determine if ticlopidine is more beneficial than aspirin in prevention of recurrent stroke in African-American patients, since it appeared more effective than aspirin in preventing stroke in African-American patients with TIA.[47]

All patients with a history of ischemic stroke without contraindications should receive lifelong antiplatelet therapy with aspirin or clopidogrel. In patients intolerant to aspirin or who experience an event while on aspirin, clopidogrel or ticlopidine should be considered, although clopidogrel is preferred based on its better safety and tolerability profile.

Acute Therapy of the Brain Attack
Intravenous Thrombolytic Therapy

For the first time, a therapy for acute ischemic stroke can actually improve the outcome of patients and reverse some neurologic deficits. In the NIH trial, intravenous administration of tPA within 3 hours of the onset of stroke symptoms increased the number of patients with a 'good outcome' at 3-month follow-up, from 21% in patients treated with placebo to 31% in patients treated with tPA.[48] tPA is infused at 0.9 mg/kg over 1 hour, with 10% given as a bolus injection, up to a maximum of 90 mg. 'Good outcome' was measured with functional scales (Barthel index and Rankin), which established the ability of the patient to perform activities of daily living. Only patients with normal or near-normal function were classified as 'good outcome.' Another thrombolytic agent, streptokinase (Streptase®), was evaluated in three clinical trials, but is not used because of an unacceptable level of adverse outcomes from intracerebral hemorrhage.[49-51]

A statistically significant benefit of treatment with tPA was only demonstrable at 3-month follow-up; no significant beneficial effect was documented 24 hours or 7 days after administration. This is related to the hemorrhagic complications of tPA. Hemorrhagic transformation of infarction occurred in 6.4% of the treated patients and in only 0.6% of the placebo patients. The acute mortality rate for tPA treatment was 3.6%. However, the overall mortality rate after 3 months was equal in treated and untreated patients. This suggests that patients with large infarctions are at risk of dying acutely with administration of tPA, but that these same types of patients ultimately succumb to the medical complications of severe stroke during the subsequent 3 months. Table 1 lists guidelines for administration of tPA.

Before administration of tPA, the clinician must document that the patient has had a stroke within 3 hours; that CT scan shows no hemorrhagic component to the stroke; and that the mean arterial blood pressure is not above 130 mm Hg. tPA cannot be administered to patients who have had surgical procedures within 1 week, who are taking warfarin, who have an elevated PT or PTT, or who have thrombocytopenia or any other predisposition to hemorrhage. Patients with severe stroke (NIH stroke scale >22) and patients over age 77 have a higher risk of poor outcome secondary to hemorrhage.

The difficulties associated with administration of tPA to acute stroke patients are demonstrated in the European Cooperative Acute Stroke Study (ECASS).[52] In the ECASS trial, treatment with tPA or placebo had an equal number of good and poor outcomes, with severe hemorrhagic complications outweighing any beneficial effects of thrombolysis. The ECASS trial and the NIH trial of tPA had several differences, however. The time window for treatment with tPA was up to 6 hours, rather than 3 hours in the ECASS trial. Heparin and aspirin could be administered after tPA infusion whereas, in the NIH trial, they could not be administered for 24 hours after infusion. Analysis of the patients with hemorrhagic complications in the ECASS trial identified a subset of patients with early changes of infarction seen on CT brain scan involving more than one third of the affected cerebral hemisphere.[53] The signs of subtle hemorrhage or early infarction are often difficult to identify on CT, and a skilled neuroradiologist or neurologist must examine the scan before administration of tPA[54] (Figure 4).

Although thrombolytic therapy with tPA was shown to be effective in improving outcome of stroke patients in the NIH trial, clinical judgment is still necessary for determining the appropriateness of administration of tPA in each individual patient. Further evaluation of the efficacy of tPA using a 6-hour window did not show a significant benefit in the primary outcome of functional capacity measured by the modified Rankin scale at 90 days after treatment.[55] Analysis of secondary endpoints did show a trend toward a benefit of tPA treatment.[56] The results of the study emphasized the importance of clinical judgment in the appropriate use of tPA in each case.[55-57] A more recent study found no beneficial effect of administering tPA between 3 and 5 hours after stroke because of the high incidence of cerebral hemorrhage.[58]

Table 1: Guidelines for Administration of Intravenous tPA

Inclusion Criteria

- Age: 18-85
- Clinical diagnosis of ischemic stroke with onset of symptoms within 3 hours of initiation of therapy
- Noncontrast head CT without evidence of hemorrhage

Exclusion Criteria

- Stroke or head trauma within the past 3 months
- Major surgery, gastrointestinal or genitourinary bleeding within the past 2 weeks
- History of intracranial hemorrhage or bleeding disorder
- Arterial puncture at noncompressible site within the past week
- Deep coma/stupor
- Pregnancy
- Mild stroke or improving deficit
- Persistent elevation of blood pressure despite treatment (systolic >185; diastolic >110)
- Recent myocardial infarction
- Recent lumbar puncture
- Platelet count <100,000
- Elevated prothrombin time (PT) >15 seconds
- Elevated partial thromboplastin time (PTT) on heparin therapy
- Blood glucose <40 or >400
- CT evidence of early irreversible infarction involving more than one third of a cerebral hemisphere

Protocol
- Apply cardiac monitor
- Apply oxygen therapy
- Place intravenous and draw stat CBC, platelets, PT/PTT, blood type, and cross match in case transfusion is necessary
- Emergency evaluation by stroke neurologist
- Emergency noncontrast CT scan of brain, read by radiologist and/or neurologist
- Initiate thrombolytic therapy if all procedures are completed within 3 hours after onset of symptoms

tPA Administration
- 0.9 mg/kg to a maximum of 90 mg
- 10% of total dose is given as an IV bolus
- Remainder of dose at a constant infusion over the next 60 minutes
- Blood pressure maintained below 185/110, monitor every 15 minutes
- No aspirin, heparin, or warfarin for the next 24 hours

Guidelines for the administration of intravenous tissue plasminogen activator (recombinant alteplase, Activase®) derived from:

Adams HP Jr, Brott TG, Furlan AJ, et al: Guidelines for thrombolytic therapy for acute stroke: a supplement to the guidelines for the management of patients with acute ischemic stroke. A statement for healthcare professionals from a Special Writing Group of the Stroke Council, American Heart Association. *Circulation* 1996;94:1167-1174.

Quality Standards Subcommittee of the American Academy of Neurology: Practice advisory: thrombolytic therapy for acute ischemic stroke—summary statement. *Neurology* 1996;47:835-839.

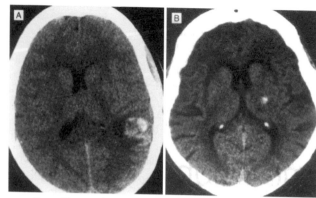

Easy Hemorrhage:
24 of 24 (100%)

Difficult Hemorrhage:
25 of 33 (76%)

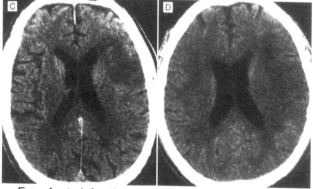

Easy Acute Infarction:
17 of 21 (81%)

Intermediate Acute Infarction:
23 of 43 (53%)

Figure 4: *The signs of cerebral hemorrhage and infarction on CT scan of the brain that contraindicate the use of rt-tPA. An easily detectable hemorrhage (A), subtle hemorrhage (B), easily detectable infarction (C), and subtle infarction (D) are shown. The frequency of correct interpretation of each of these scans by a group of neurologists and neuroradiologists is shown.[54] Used with permission.*

Some controversy exists whether tPA is as effective as it appeared in the NIH trial, since the patients with lacunar stroke in the placebo group had a more severe disability at entry than did the patients in the treated group. This may have contributed to the favorable outcome of administration of tPA to patients with lacunar stroke.[59] Some experts are calling for further trials to delineate which patients benefit most from tPA therapy, so that patients for whom treatment is not applicable will not be exposed to the risk of hemorrhage.[60]

The greatest drawback to intravenous thrombolytic therapy is that it must be administered within 3 hours of onset of acute stroke symptoms. Only 1% to 6% of patients with acute stroke arrive at the hospital in time to be eligible for tPA.[61] This is partly because many patients arise in the morning with stroke symptoms, and the time of night the actual stroke occurred cannot be documented. However, a large proportion of patients and medical professionals are not aware that an acute therapy for stroke is available, and, thus, patients do not arrive at the hospital in time for treatment. Public education about the necessity of obtaining acute treatment for a brain attack may be the most important advance in therapy of acute ischemic stroke.

Intra-Arterial Thrombolytic Therapy

Thrombolytic agents can be administered directly into an occluded or stenotic cerebral artery during the course of cerebral angiography, typically within 6 hours after onset of ischemic stroke, although the procedure for administering the intra-arterial thrombolytic agent may take several hours. Anecdotal reports describe reestablishing patency of occluded cerebral and vertebrobasilar arteries with direct intra-arterial urokinase and tPA, with clinical improvement in some instances, but a high risk of hemorrhage.[62-64]

A randomized trial of intra-arterial recombinant pro-urokinase (rpro-UK) (Prolyse) versus placebo was performed in patients with middle cerebral artery occlusion.[65] Among 105 patients who underwent angiography, rpro-UK was administered to 26 and placebo to 14 within a median of 5.5 hours from onset of symptoms. A dose of 6 mg/kg of rpro-UK was administered over 120 minutes into the proximal end of the thrombus. All patients received intravenous heparin for 4 hours, 16 received a 100-unit/kg bolus followed by a 1,000 unit/h constant infusion (high heparin), and 24 received a 2,000-unit bolus followed by a 500-unit/h infusion (low heparin). In the high-heparin group, partial to complete recanalization occurred in 81.8% of 11 patients treated with rpro-UK, compared with 0 of 5 patients treated with placebo. In the low-heparin group, recanalization occurred in 40% of 15 patients treated with rpro-UK and 22.2% of 9 placebo patients. Recanalization was statistically significant in the high-heparin group treated with rpro-UK, but this group had a 72.7% incidence of cerebral hemorrhage, 27.3% with clinical deterioration. The overall incidence of hemorrhage was 50.0% in the treated group (15.4% with deterioration) and 35.7% in the placebo group (14.3% with clinical deterioration). The overall number of good outcomes as determined by the Barthel index and modified Rankin scores was equivalent in treated and placebo patients.

A subsequent study in 180 patients with middle cerebral artery occlusion showed a beneficial effect of intra-arterial administration of 9 mg rpro-UK with heparin 6 hours after stroke. A favorable outcome occurred (modified Rankin score of 2 or less) in 40% of 121 patients treated with rpro-UK and 27% of 59 control patients treated only with heparin ($P=0.04$). The recanalization rate was 66% for the rpro-UK group and 19% for the control group ($P<0.0001$). The risk of symptomatic intracranial hemorrhage was 10% in the rpro-UK patients and 2% on the control patients ($P<0.06$).[66]

A trial of rpro-UK, 9 mg/kg, is under way to determine if greater clinical improvement is possible. However, intra-arterial thrombolysis cannot be recommended except possibly in the instance of progressive basilar artery occlusion in a patient with progressive obtundation, in whom the outcome is expected to be so grave that the risk of hemorrhagic complication is acceptable.[64]

Hypervolemic Hemodilution

Researchers have attempted to increase cerebral perfusion in ischemic stroke with hypervolemic hemodilution. Previous studies employing low-molecular-weight dextrans[67] and a recent study employing 10% hydroxyethyl starch have not been effective when compared to rehydration alone.[68]

Neuroprotective Agents

Experimental studies in animal models of ischemia have identified several agents that can prevent ischemic neuronal damage, particularly inhibitors of the NMDA receptor, which allows for calcium influx into neurons when stimulated by excitotoxic neurotransmitters.[69] However, in human studies, many of these agents caused unacceptable side effects in phase I trials, and the agents that proceeded to randomized controlled trials (Selfotel, Aptiganel) have not been found to have a beneficial effect.

An agent that inhibits glutamate release, lubeluzole, has shown a small beneficial effect in one trial compared to placebo when given within 6 hours after stroke,[70] but did not have a beneficial effect in another.[71] The inhibitory neurotransmitter gamma-aminobutyric acid (GABA) counteracts the effects of excitotoxic neurotransmitters in vivo, and although a GABA-mimetic agent, clomethiazole, was not successful overall, patients with large cortical infarctions in the middle cerebral artery territory appeared to benefit, prompting a further trial in this subgroup of patients.[72] The excitatory neurotransmitter glycine potentiates the activity of the NMDA receptor, and a glycine antagonist, GV150526, has completed phase II trial. A phase III randomized trial is being undertaken to determine effectiveness.[73]

Inhibition of calcium influx with the voltage-gated L-N channel inhibitor nimodipine (Nimotop®) did not show improvement in outcome when administered in a time window of 24 to 48 hours,[74] but may have had some benefit in patients who received the drug within 12 hours.[75] A clinical trial with a 6-hour time window is under way.[59]

Prevention of reperfusion injury by limiting lipid peroxidation is another important consideration in treatment of ischemic stroke, particularly in cardioembolic stroke and in patients who receive thrombolytic therapy. A trial of the antioxidant tirilazad mesylate, a 21-aminosteroid, has not been successful in improving outcome in ischemic stroke.[76] An intercellular adhesion monoclonal antibody (ICAM) has been used to inhibit entry of neutrophils into zones of ischemic infarction to reduce oxidative stress, but was not successful in clinical trials.[77] A membrane-stabilizing agent, citicoline, had shown some promise for improving outcome in two randomized trials,[78,79] but a recent, more definitive trial was terminated because of lack of successful outcome.

Stroke in Young Adults

In patients under age 45, arteriosclerotic etiologies of stroke are less common, and other sources of stroke predominate. In a recent series of 428 stroke patients under age 45, 31.1% were caused by cardiogenic embolism, 19.8% by hematologic abnormalities, 19.8% by lacunar infarctions (from hypertension and diabetes), 11.3% by nonatherosclerotic vasculopathy, 9.4% by illicit drug use, 5.2% by oral contraceptive use, only 3.8% by large-artery atherosclerotic disease, and 1.4% by complicated migraine.[80] No probable or possible cause of stroke could be identified in 31.8% of these patients. Among the cardioembolic group, endocarditis, prosthetic heart valve, cardiomyopathy or akinetic wall, and intracardiac thrombus predominated. Mitral valve prolapse also was implicated as a probable cause of stroke when no other source could be determined.

Nonatherosclerotic vasculopathy and hematologic causes included eclampsia and preeclampsia associated with pregnancy, in which uncontrolled hypertension is the main factor and is treated with antihypertensive medications.[81]

In the postpartum period, venous sinus or cortical vein thrombosis can occur. Cerebral infarction with focal neurologic deficits can be caused by the venous obstruction, and hemorrhage also can occur.[82] Patients often present with headache and fever in addition to the symptoms of stroke. Increased intracranial pressure with papilledema may be present. The radiologic diagnosis often is difficult, but can be made on CT scan of the brain if a 'delta sign' appears in the region of the confluens of venous sinuses. Magnetic resonance venography can help establish diagnosis, but cerebral angiography sometimes is necessary. Even with the risk of hemorrhagic complications, heparin is recommended to prevent spread of the thrombosis. Retrograde intravenous administration of urokinase also has been used to resolve venous thrombosis.[83] When intracranial pressure is elevated, corticosteroids and mannitol are used.

Cerebral venous thrombosis can also cause cerebral infarction in patients with lupus erythematosus. However, the main sources of stroke in patients with lupus are cardioembolic, including emboli from Libman-Sacks endocarditis.[84] In lupus patients, thrombotic thrombocytopenic purpura can cause both infarction from occlusion of vessels by platelets and hemorrhage from the thrombocytopenia. Inflammatory vasculitis in patients with lupus erythematosus is exceedingly rare, and is more common in polyarteritis nodosa.[85] However, lupus patients have a hyaline vasculopathy,[85] which can cause reduction in focal and global cerebral blood flow.[86,87] A hypercoagulable state also may be associated with the presence of the anticardiolipin antibody or lupus anticoagulant, which can occur without other manifestations of systemic lupus, and should be addressed in all young stroke patients.[88] Treatment of cerebrovascular disease associated with lupus includes anti-inflammatory agents such as corticosteroids, anticoagulation with heparin in patients in a thrombotic state or with intracardiac thrombosis, and management of platelet disorders.

A primary granulomatous angiitis of the central nervous system that is not associated with other collagen-vascular disease also may occur, and can cause focal infarction or hemorrhage.[89] The diagnosis can be made by cerebral angiography and biopsy of the leptomeningeal vessels. The usual treatment is corticosteroids. Takayasu's disease is a giant cell arteritis of the great vessels emanating from the aorta, which can cause occlusion of the common carotid or internal carotid arteries, with resultant cerebral infarction.[90] Occlusion of the intracranial internal carotid artery can occur in moyamoya disease, whose etiology is not clear.[91] Hemorrhagic complications can occur in moyamoya disease; therefore, anticoagulation is used only in patients with progressive ischemic symptoms. A vasculopathy also can occur as a complication of intravenous drug use, particularly cocaine, which can result in infarction or hemorrhage.[92]

Stroke is a major complication of sickle cell anemia in children and young adults. During a sickle crisis, inspissation of erythrocytes can injure the endothelium of large vessels, causing thrombosis of the internal carotid artery and large branches such as the middle cerebral artery.[93] Therapy with exchange transfusion can restore circulation and prevent further vascular occlusions, but must be done on a prophylactic basis in at-risk patients.[93] Transcranial Doppler ultrasound was recently used to identify sickle cell patients with vascular occlusive disease on routine screening before onset of stroke, and a study is under way to determine if prophylactic exchange transfusion is useful in preventing stroke in these patients.[94]

Migraine

Migraine is thought to be induced by vasospasm, and may be equivalent to coronary vasospasm causing angina and myocardial infarction. The initial vasoconstrictive component appears to be initiated by serotonin (5-hydroxytryptamine or 5-HT), which is thought to be released from platelets.[95] A prodrome of scintillating visual scotomata and nausea occurs in classic migraine, followed by throbbing hemicranial headache from compensatory vasodilation, which can last for several hours.[96] Focal neurologic deficits can occur in this prodromal phase of migraine and sometimes last for hours or days, occasionally becoming irreversible if ischemia is sufficient to cause infarction.[97] In these patients, ergot alkaloids such as Cafergot or the 5-HT receptor blockers such as sumatriptan (Imitrex®) are contraindicated because they can exacerbate ischemic symptoms.[98-101] Daily prophylactic therapy is needed in patients with complicated migraine. Inhibition of platelet aggregation with aspirin to reduce serotonin release has had limited success.[98] Vasodilators, including the β-adrenergic blockers propranolol (Inderal®) 40 to 240 mg q.d. and atenolol 20 to 60 mg q.d., have been used, but can worsen ischemia if an attack occurs because of decreased perfusion from hypotension.[98] Calcium-channel blockers in the verapamil family, such as Calan® 120 to 240 mg/d, have been effective in many cases.[98] The most successful agent has been the serotonin antagonist methysergide (Sansert®), but this can be administered only in the most extreme conditions and for a limited time because of the complication of retroperitoneal fibrosis.[101,102]

Management of Patients After Stroke

The most significant factor for management of post-stroke patients is prevention of recurrent stroke. The measures instituted in the initial evaluation of the stroke patient to prevent further stroke should be continued. Rehabilitation therapy is beneficial in enabling the stroke

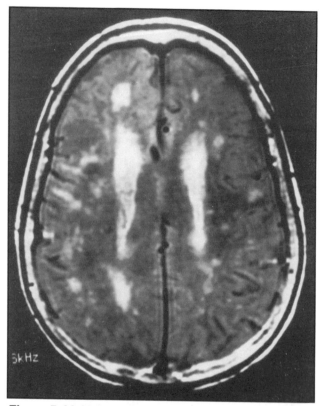

5kHz

Figure 5: *Multiple small areas of infarction and ischemic changes in white matter (leukoariosis) are seen in white in this T2-weighted MRI from a patient with multi-infarct dementia. Courtesy of Dr. Adam Silvers.*

patient to achieve as much independence as possible in activities of daily living by teaching the patient alternative strategies to accomplish tasks, as well as by improvement of function of affected structures.

Early rehabilitation intervention can prevent contractures of spastic extremities, which can be painful as well as disabling. Pharmacologic agents to counteract spasticity, such as baclofen and dantrolene (Dantrium®), have not been very successful in stroke patients, and reducing the spasticity of a lower extremity can actually reduce the potential for weight bearing and ambulation. Gait training and provision of appropriate prosthetic devices, such as a quad cane or walker, can enable the patient to recover ambulation. Recent experimental trials with local injection of botulinum toxin into spastic upper extremity muscles have shown reduction in spasticity, but are still in progress to determine if function is improved.

Poststroke depression occurs in 25% to 33% of stroke patients, mainly after dominant hemisphere infarctions in the frontal lobe. It can diminish the patient's functional capacity.[103-106] Pharmacologic treatment of depression with agents that enhance catecholaminergic function (eg, amitriptyline [Elavil®], imipramine [Tofranil®]) has been successful.[107] Serotonergic agents such as fluoxetine (Prozac®), paroxetine (Paxil®), and sertraline (Zoloft®) are also used. Occasionally, electroconvulsive shock therapy is necessary, particularly when a patient is too depressed to eat. However, this can have complications in patients with organic deficits.

Poststroke pain can occur secondary to spasticity. A paretic arm can also become painful from reflex neurovascular dystrophy, also known as the shoulder-hand syndrome.[108] Painful swelling occurs in the hand and shoulder, followed by contractures of the joints and atrophic changes of the skin and muscles. When severe, it is treated with sympathetic blockade of the upper extremity.[108] Lesions involving the thalamus also can cause a painful dysesthesia on the contralateral face and body, starting 3 to 6 months after stroke.[109] This central neurogenic pain usually responds to anticonvulsive medications such as carbamazepine (Tegretol®) or gabapentin (Neurontin®), often used in combination with antidepressant medications such as amitriptyline or fluoxetine.

Cognitive deficits after stroke are common,[110] even when a patient appears to be fully recovered from any focal motor or sensory deficits. A minor language deficit can interfere with cognitive function, and speech therapy should be considered. Focal lesions in the cingulate gyrus can cause apathy that can mimic a generalized dementia. Specific deficits in memory and recall can be caused by infarction in the hippocampus or medial thalamus.[111] Lesions in the angular gyrus and limbic system of the medial temporal lobe can cause abnormal emotional behavior similar to Alzheimer's disease.[111] A cerebral infarction can exacerbate the cognitive dysfunction of patients with coexisting Alzheimer's disease. Multiple small infarctions can cause multi-infarct dementia (Figure 5). These cognitive factors must be accounted for in discharge planning and rehabilitative strategies.

Conclusion

The treatment of acute stroke is now grounded on a firm scientific basis. The timing and methods of anticoagulant and antiplatelet therapy have clear indications. The introduction of thrombolytic therapy opened a new vista in the treatment of acute stroke as a brain attack. New strategies using neuroprotective agents are being developed to reduce the extent of ischemic damage. The greatest promise seems to lie in a combination of thrombolytic therapy to restore cerebral perfusion, combined with neuroprotective agents that can salvage ischemic neurons and prevent reperfusion injury. However, patients, physicians, and emergency service workers must be educated about the concept of the brain attack to maximize the benefit that stroke patients may achieve from the advances in thrombolytic therapy.

The future of therapy for ischemic stroke appears promising, but further work must be done. Even though we have a greater understanding of the mechanisms of stroke and strategies for preventing stroke by control of risk factors, the dramatic decline in stroke mortality achieved in the 1970s has not continued, and stroke continues to be the third leading cause of death in the United States.[112]

References

1.   Komrad MS, Coffey CE, Coffey KS, et al: Myocardial infarction and stroke. *Neurology* 1984;34:1403-1409.

2.   Asinger RW, Mikell FL, Elsperger J, et al: Incidence of left-ventricular thrombosis after acute transmural myocardial infarction. Serial evaluation by two-dimensional echocardiography. *N Engl J Med* 1981;305:297-302.

3.   Melville KI, Shister HE: Cardiac responses to epinephrine and norepinephrine during prolonged cholesterol and high fat feeding in rabbits. *Am J Cardiol* 1959;4:391-400.

4.   Myers MG, Norris JW, Hachinski VC, et al: Cardiac sequelae of acute stroke. *Stroke* 1982;13:838-842.

5.   Mikolich JR, Jacobs WC, Fletcher GF: Cardiac arrhythmias in patients with acute cerebrovascular accidents. *JAMA* 1981; 246:1314-1317.

6.   Oppenheimer SM, Cechetto DF, Hachinski VC: Cerebrogenic cardiac arrhythmias. Cerebral electrocardiographic influences and their role in sudden death. *Arch Neurol* 1990;47:513-519.

7.   Lavy S, Yaar I, Melamed E, et al: The effect of acute stroke on cardiac functions as observed in an intensive stroke care unit. *Stroke* 1974;5:775-780.

8.   Wallace JD, Levy LL: Blood pressure after stroke. *JAMA* 1981;246:2177-2180.

9.   Astrup J, Siesjo BK, Symon L: Thresholds in cerebral ischemia—the ischemic penumbra. *Stroke* 1981;12:723-725.

10.   Pulsinelli W, Waldman S, Sigsbee B, et al: Experimental hyperglycemia and diabetes mellitus worsen stroke outcome. *Trans Am Neurol Assoc* 1980;105:21-24.

11.   Ginsberg MD, Welsh FA, Budd WW: Deleterious effect of glucose pretreatment on recovery from diffuse cerebral ischemia in the cat. I. Local cerebral blood flow and glucose utilization. *Stroke* 1980;11:347-354.

12.   Welsh FA, Ginsberg MD, Rieder W, et al: Deleterious effect of glucose pretreatment on recovery from diffuse cerebral ischemia in the cat. II. Regional metabolite levels. *Stroke* 1980;11:355-363.

13. Weinberger J, Biscarra V, Weisberg MK, et al: Factors contributing to stroke in patients with atherosclerotic disease of the great vessels: the role of diabetes. *Stroke* 1983;14:709-712.

14. Woo J, Lam CW, Kay R, et al: The influence of hyperglycemia and diabetes mellitus on immediate and 3-month morbidity and mortality after acute stroke. *Arch Neurol* 1990;47:1174-1177.

15. Axelsson K, Asplund K, Norberg A, et al: Nutritional status in patients with acute stroke. *Acta Med Scand* 1988;224:217-224.

16. Bounds JV, Wiebers DO, Whisnant JP, et al: Mechanisms and timing of deaths from cerebral infarction. *Stroke* 1981;12:474-477.

17. Theodore J, Robin ED: Pathogenesis of neurogenic pulmonary oedema. *Lancet* 1975;2:749-751.

18. Patten BM, Mendell J, Bruun B, et al: Double-blind study of the effects of dexamethasone on acute stroke. *Neurology* 1972; 22:377-383.

19. Bauer RB, Tellez H: Dexamethasone as treatment in cerebrovascular disease. 2. A controlled study in acute cerebral infarction. *Stroke* 1973;4:547-555.

20. Mathew NT, Rivera VM, Meyer JS, et al: Double-blind evaluation of glycerol therapy in acute cerebral infarction. *Lancet* 1972;2:1327-1329.

21. Schwab S, Hacke W: Therapy of increased intracranial pressure in space-occupying media infarcts. *Z Arztl Fortbild Qualitatssich* 1999;93(3):203-208.

22. Schwab S, Schwarz S, Bertram M, et al: Moderate hypothermia for the treatment of malignant middle cerebral artery infarct. *Nervenarzt* 1999;70(6):539-546.

23. Schwab S, Steiner S, Aschoff A, et al: Early hemicraniectomy in patients with complete middle cerebral artery infarction. *Stroke* 1999;29(9):1888-1893.

24. Kilpatrick CJ, Davis SM, Tress BM, et al: Epileptic seizures in acute stroke. *Arch Neurol* 1990;47:157-160.

25. Gupta SR, Naheedy MH, Elias D, et al: Postinfarction seizures. A clinical study. *Stroke* 1988;19:1477-1481.

26. Haley EC Jr, Kassell NF, Torner JC: Failure of heparin to prevent progression in progressing ischemic infarction. *Stroke* 1988;19:10-14.

27. Duke RJ, Bloch RF, Turpie AG, et al: Intravenous heparin for the prevention of stroke progression in acute partial stable stroke. *Ann Intern Med* 1986;105:825-828.

28. Baker RN, Broward JA, Fang HC, et al: Anticoagulant therapy in cerebral infarction. Report on cooperative study. *Neurology* 1962;12:823-830.

29. Fisher CM: The use of anticoagulants in cerebral thrombosis. *Neurology* 1958;8:311-332.

30. Liu J, Tuhrim S, Weinberger J, et al: Premonitory symptoms of stroke in evolution to the locked-in state. *J Neurol Neurosurg Psychiatry* 1983;46:221-226.

31. The Publications Committee for the Trial of ORG 10172 in Acute Stroke Treatment (TOAST) Investigators: Low molecular weight heparinoid, ORG 10172 (danaparoid), and outcome after acute ischemic stroke: a randomized controlled trial. *JAMA* 1998;279:1265-1272.

32. Adams HP Jr, Bendixen BH, Leira E, et al: Antithrombotic treatment of ischemic stroke among patients with occlusion or severe stenosis of the internal carotid artery: A report of the Trial of Org 10172 in Acute Stroke Treatment (TOAST). *Neurology* 1999;53:122-125.

33. Kay R, Wong KS, Yu YL, et al: Low-molecular-weight heparin for the treatment of acute ischemic stroke. *N Engl J Med* 1995;333:1588-1593.

34. International Stroke Trial Collaborative Group: The International Stroke Trial (IST): a randomised trial of aspirin, subcutaneous heparin, both, or neither among 19435 patients with acute ischaemic stroke. *Lancet* 1997;349:1569-1581.

35. Fisher CM, Ojemann RG, Roberson GH: Spontaneous dissection of cervico-cerebral arteries. *Can J Neurol Sci* 1978;5:9-19.

36. Hart RG: Vertebral artery dissection. *Neurology* 1988;38:987-989.

37. Weinberger J, Rudolph S, Lidov M: Evidence for arterial embolization in dissecting aneurysm of the cervical vertebral artery. *J Stroke Cerebrovasc Dis* 1991;1:95-97.

38. Koller RL: Recurrent embolic cerebral infarction and anticoagulation. *Neurology* 1982;32:283-285.

39. Cerebral Embolism Study Group: Immediate anticoagulation of embolic stroke: a randomized trial. *Stroke* 1983;14:668-676.

40. Cerebral Embolism Study Group: Immediate anticoagulation of embolic stroke: brain hemorrhage and management options. *Stroke* 1984;15:779-789.

41. Rothrock JF, Dittrich HC, McAllen S, et al: Acute anticoagulation following cardioembolic stroke. *Stroke* 1989;20:730-734.

42. Pessin MS, Estol CJ, Lafranchise F, et al: Safety of anticoagulation after hemorrhagic infarction. *Neurology* 1993; 43:1298-1303.

43. Pruitt AA, Rubin RH, Karchmer AW, et al: Neurologic complications of bacterial endocarditis. *Medicine (Baltimore)* 1978; 57:329-343.

44. Chimowitz MI, Kokkinos J, Strong J, et al: The Warfarin-Aspirin Symptomatic Intracranial Disease Study. *Neurology* 1995;45:1488-1493.

45. Gent M, Blakely JA, Easton JD, et al: The Canadian American Ticlopidine Study (CATS) in thromboembolic stroke. *Lancet* 1989;1:1215-1220.

46. CAPRIE Steering Committee: A randomised, blinded trial of clopidogrel versus aspirin in patients at risk of ischaemic events (CAPRIE). *Lancet* 1996;348:1329-1339.

47. Hass WK, Easton JD, Adams HP Jr, et al: A randomized trial comparing ticlopidine hydrochloride with aspirin for the prevention of stroke in high-risk patients. Ticlopidine Aspirin Stroke Study Group. *N Engl J Med* 1988;321:501-507.

48. The National Institute of Neurological Disorders and Stroke rt-PA Stroke Study Group: Tissue plasminogen activator for acute ischemic stroke. *N Engl J Med* 1995;333:1581-1587.

49. Multicentre Acute Stroke Trial—Italy (MAST-I) Group: Randomised controlled trial of streptokinase, aspirin, and combination of both in treatment of acute ischaemic stroke. *Lancet* 1995;346:1509-1514.

50. Donnan GA, Davis SM, Chambers BR, et al: Streptokinase for acute ischemic stroke with relationship to time of administration: Australian Streptokinase (ASK) Trial Study Group. *JAMA* 1996;276:961-966.

51. The Multicenter Acute Stroke Trial—Europe Study Group: Thrombolytic therapy with streptokinase in acute ischemic stroke. *N Engl J Med* 1996;335:145-150.

52. Hacke W, Kaste M, Fieschi C, et al: Intravenous thrombolysis with recombinant tissue plasminogen activator for acute hemispheric stroke. The European Cooperative Acute Stroke Study. *JAMA* 1995;274:1017-1025.

53. Wolpert SM, Bruckmann H, Greenlee R, et al: Neuroradiologic evaluation of patients with acute stroke treated with recombinant tissue plasminogen activator. The rt-PA Acute Stroke Study Group. *AJNR Am J Neuroradiol* 1993;14:3-13.

54. Schriger DL, Kalafut M, Starkman S, et al: Cranial computed tomography interpretation in acute stroke: physician accuracy in determining eligibility for thrombolytic therapy. *JAMA* 1998; 279:1293-1297.

55. Hacke W, Kaste M, Fieschi C, et al: Randomised double-blind placebo-controlled trial of thrombolytic therapy with intravenous alteplase in acute ischaemic stroke (ECASS II). Second European-Australasian Acute Stroke Study Investigators. *Lancet* 1998;352:1245-1251.

56. Hacke W, Bluhmki E, Steiner T, et al: Dichotomized efficacy end points and global end-point analysis applied to the ECASS intention-to-treat data set: post hoc analysis of ECASS I. *Stroke* 1998;29(10):2073-2075.

57. Boysen G, Vostrup S, Bogousslavsky J: Thrombolysis for stroke: time for a consensus. *Cerebrovasc Dis* 1996;6:376-380.

58. Clark WM, Wissman S, Albers GW, et al: Recombinant tissue-type plasminogen activator (Alteplase) for ischemic stroke 3 to 5 hours after symptom onset. The ATLANTIS Study: a randomized controlled trial. *JAMA* 1999;282:2019-2026.

59. Fisher M, Bogousslavsky J: Further evolution toward effective therapy for acute ischemic stroke. *JAMA* 1998;279:1298-1303.

60. Caplan LR, Mohr JP, Kistler JP, et al: Should thrombolytic therapy be the first-line treatment for acute ischemic stroke? Thrombolysis—not a panacea for ischemic stroke. *N Engl J Med* 1997; 337:1309-1310.

61. Overgaard K, Sereghy T, Pedersen H, et al: Effect of delayed thrombolysis with rt-PA in a rat embolic stroke model. *J Cereb Blood Flow Metab* 1994;14:472-477.

62.   Fletcher AP, Alkjaersig N, Lewis M, et al: A pilot study of urokinase therapy in cerebral infarction. *Stroke* 1976;7:135-142.

63.   Theron J, Courtheoux P, Casasco A, et al: Local intraarterial fibrinolysis in the carotid territory. *AJNR Am J Neuroradiol* 1989;10:753-765.

64.   Zeumer H, Hacke W, Ringelstein EB: Local intraarterial thrombolysis in vertebrobasilar thromboembolic disease. *AJNR Am J Neuroradiol* 1983;4:401-404.

65.   del Zoppo GJ, Higashida RT, Furlan AJ, et al: PROACT: a phase II randomized trial of recombinant pro-urokinase by direct arterial delivery in acute middle cerebral artery stroke. PROACT Investigators. Prolyse in Acute Cerebral Thromboembolism. *Stroke* 1998;29:4-11.

66.   Furlan A, Higashida R, Wechler L, et al: Intra-arterial Prourokinase for acute ischemic stroke. The PROACT II Study: a randomized control trial. *JAMA* 1999;282:2003-2011.

67.   Scandinavian Stroke Study Group: Multicenter trial of hemodilution in ischemic stroke. I. Results in the total patient population. *Stroke* 1987;18:691-699.

68.   Aichner FT, Fazekas F, Brainin M, et al: Hypervolemic hemodilution in acute ischemic stroke: the Multicenter Austrian Hemodilution Stroke Trial (MAHST). *Stroke* 1998;29:743-749.

69.   Muir KW, Lees KR: Clinical experience with excitatory amino acid antagonist drugs. *Stroke* 1995;26:503-513.

70.   Grotta J: Lubeluzole treatment of acute ischemic stroke. The US and Canadian Lubeluzole Ischemic Stroke Study Group. *Stroke* 1997;28:2338-2346.

71.   Diener HC, Kaste M, Hacke W, et al: Lubeluzole in acute ischemic stroke. *Stroke* 1997;28:271.

72.   Wahlgren NG, Bognhov S, Sharma A, et al: The Clomethiazole Acute Stroke Study (CLASS). Efficacy results in 545 patients classified as total anterior circulation syndrome. *J Stroke Cardiovasc Dis* 1999;8:231-239.

73.   GAIN Investigators: Phase II studies of the glycine antagonist, GV 150526, in acute stroke (GAIN). *Stroke* 1998;29:304.

74.   Silver B, Weber J, Fisher M: Medical therapy for ischemic stroke. *Clin Neuropharmacol* 1996;19:101-128.

75. Mohr JP, Orgogozo JM, Harrison MJ, et al: Meta-analysis of oral nimodipine trials in acute ischemic stroke. *Cerebrovasc Dis* 1994;4:197-203.

76. The RANTTAS Investigators: A randomized trial of tirilazad mesylate in patients with acute stroke (RANTTAS). *Stroke* 1996;27:1453-1458.

77. The Enlimolab Acute Stroke Trial Investigators: The Enlimolab Acute Stroke Trial: final results [abstract]. *Neurology* 1997;48.

78. Clark WM, Warach SJ, Pettigrew LC, et al: A randomized dose-response trial of citicoline in acute ischemic stroke. *Neurology* 1997;49:671-678.

79. Clark WM, Williams BJ, Selzer KA, et al: Randomized efficacy trial of citicoline in acute ischemic stroke [abstract]. *Stroke* 1998;29:287.

80. Kittner SJ, Stern BJ, Wozniak M, et al: Cerebral infarction in young adults: the Baltimore-Washington Cooperative Young Stroke Study. *Neurology* 1998;50:890-894.

81. Kittner SJ, Stern BJ, Feeser BR, et al: Pregnancy and risk of stroke. *N Engl J Med* 1996;335:768-774.

82. Bousser MG, Chiras J, Bories J, et al: Cerebral venous thrombosis—a review of 38 cases. *Stroke* 1985;16:199-213.

83. Horowitz M, Purdy P, Unwin H, et al: Treatment of dural sinus thrombosis using selective catheterization and urokinase. *Ann Neurol* 1995;38:58-67.

84. Devinsky O, Petito CK, Alonso DR: Clinical and neuropathological findings in systemic lupus erythematosus: the role of vasculitis, heart emboli, and thrombotic thrombocytopenic purpura. *Ann Neurol* 1988;23:380-384.

85. Johnson RT, Richardson EP: The neurological manifestations of systemic lupus erythematosus. *Medicine (Baltimore)* 1968; 47:337-369.

86. Weinberger J, Gordon J, Hodson AK, et al: Effect of intracerebral vasculitis on regional cerebral blood flow. *Arch Neurol* 1979;36:681-685.

87. Colamussi P, Giganti M, Cittanti C, et al: Brain single-photon emission tomography with 99mTc-HMPAO in neuropsychiatric systemic lupus erythematosus: relations with EEG and MRI findings and clinical manifestations. *Eur J Nucl Med* 1995;22:17-24.

88. The Antiphospholipid Antibodies and Stroke Study Group (APASS): Anticardiolipin antibodies and the risk of recurrent thrombo-occlusive events and death. *Neurology* 1997;48:91-94.

89. Cupps TR, Moore PM, Fauci AS: Isolated angiitis of the central nervous system. Prospective diagnostic and therapeutic experience. *Am J Med* 1983;74:97-105.

90. Ishikawa K: Natural history and classification of occlusive thromboaortopathy (Takayasu's disease). *Circulation* 1978;57:27-35.

91. Suzuki J, Takaku A: Cerebrovascular "moyamoya" disease. Disease showing abnormal net-like vessels in base of brain. *Arch Neurol* 1969;20:288-299.

92. Sloan MA, Kittner SJ, Rigamonti D, et al: Occurrence of stroke associated with use/abuse of drugs. *Neurology* 1991;41:1358-1364.

93. Russell MO, Goldberg HI, Hodson A, et al: Effect of transfusion therapy on arteriographic abnormalities and on recurrence of stroke in sickle cell disease. *Blood* 1984;63:162-169.

94. Adams RJ, McKie VC, Hsu L, et al: Prevention of a first stroke by transfusions in children with sickle cell anemia and abnormal results on transcranial Doppler ultrasonography. *N Engl J Med* 1998;339:5-11.

95. Joseph R, Welch KM: The platelet and migraine: a nonspecific association. *Headache* 1987;27:375-380.

96. Lauritzen M, Skyhoj Olsen T, Lassen NA, et al: Changes in regional cerebral blood flow during the course of classic migraine attacks. *Ann Neurol* 1983;13:633-641.

97. Rothrock JF, Walicke P, Swenson MR, et al: Migrainous stroke. *Arch Neurol* 1988;45:63-67.

98. Baumel B: Migraine: a pharmacologic review with newer options and delivery modalities. *Neurology* 1994;44:S13-S17.

99. The Subcutaneous Sumatriptan International Study Group: Treatment of migraine attacks with sumatriptan. *N Engl J Med* 1991;325:316-321.

100. Cutler N, Mushet GR, Davis R, et al: Oral sumatriptan for the acute treatment of migraine: evaluation of three dosage strengths. *Neurology* 1995;45:S5-S9.

101. Friedman AP, Elkind AH: Appraisal of methysergide in treatment of vascular headaches of migraine type. *JAMA* 1963;184:125-128.

102. Graham JR, Suby HI, LeCompte PR, et al: Fibrotic disorders associated with methysergide therapy for headache. *N Engl J Med* 1966;274:359-368.

103. Robinson RG, Starr LB, Price TR: A two year longitudinal study of mood disorders following stroke. Prevalence and duration at six months follow-up. *Br J Psychiatry* 1984;144:256-262.

104. Robinson RG, Szetela B: Mood change following left hemispheric brain injury. *Ann Neurol* 1981;9:447-453.

105. Lipsey JR, Robinson RG, Pearlson GD, et al: Mood change following bilateral hemisphere brain injury. *Br J Psychiatry* 1983;143:266-273.

106. Starkstein SE, Robinson RG, Berthier ML, et al: Differential mood changes following basal ganglia vs thalamic lesions. *Arch Neurol* 1988;45:725-730.

107. Lipsey JR, Robinson RG, Pearlson GD, et al: Nortriptyline treatment of post-stroke depression: a double-blind study. *Lancet* 1984;1:297-300.

108. Steinbrocker O, Argyros TG: The shoulder-hand syndrome: present status as a diagnostic and therapeutic entity. *Med Clin North Am* 1958;42:1533-1553.

109. Boivie J, Leijon G, Johansson I: Central post-stroke pain—a study of the mechanisms through analyses of the sensory abnormalities. *Pain* 1989;37:173-185.

110. Schut LJ: Dementia following stroke. *Clin Geriatr Med* 1988;4:767-784.

111. Tatemichi TK: How acute brain failure becomes chronic: a view of the mechanisms of dementia related to stroke. *Neurology* 1990;40:1652-1659.

112. Gillum RF, Sempos CT: The end of the long-term decline in stroke mortality in the United States? *Stroke* 1997;28:1527-1529.

Chapter **6**

Management of Hemorrhagic Stroke

Hemorrhage accounts for about 15% of strokes.[1] Of these hemorrhages, 75% are intraparenchymal hematomas, and 25% are subarachnoid bleeds.[1] Most parenchymal hemorrhages are attributable to hypertension, and involve the deep structures of the brain in the region of the basal ganglia, internal capsule, and external capsule.[2] Superficial hemorrhage into a lobe of the brain is more common in elderly patients, and is often caused

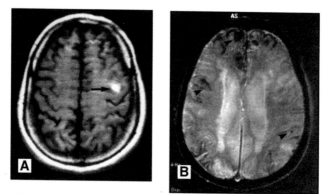

Figure 1: *(a) A small lobar hemorrhage is seen (arrow) in this T1-weighted MRI image. (b) A gradient-echo MRI revealed multiple small foci of hemosiderin deposition (arrowheads), indicating prior small hemorrhages. These findings are typical of amyloid angiopathy.*

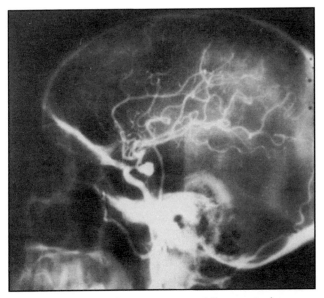

Figure 2: *A saccular aneurysm of the posterior communicating artery is demonstrated with intra-arterial contrast angiography. From: Utterback RA: Hemorrhagic cerebrovascular disease. In: Baker AB, Baker LH, eds.* Clinical Neurology. *New York, Harper & Row, 1977, chapter 11, figure 11-10. Used with permission.*

by amyloid angiopathy, which can be associated with Alzheimer's disease (Figure 1).[3] Intraparenchymal hemorrhage usually causes an acute onset of focal neurologic deficits accompanied by severe headache and progressive deterioration in level of consciousness over several minutes to hours. A significant mass effect can cause brain herniation. Secondary hemorrhages in the pons from increased intracranial pressure may complicate intracerebral hemorrhage and cause a vegetative state, even after pressure effects from the hemorrhage are reversed. Small hemorrhages may cause mild deficits and no headache,

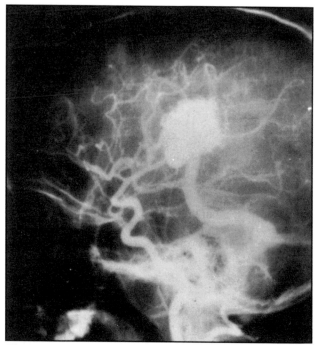

Figure 3: *An arteriovenous malformation is demonstrated with intra-arterial contrast angiography. From: Utterback RA: Hemorrhagic cerebrovascular disease. In: Baker AB, Baker LH, eds.* Clinical Neurology. *Harper & Row, 1977, chapter 11, figure 11-13. Used with permission.*

while large infarctions from internal carotid or middle cerebral artery occlusion may cause severe progressive deficits and alteration in level of consciousness. These conditions can be differentiated by computed tomography (CT) scan of the brain.

Subarachnoid hemorrhage is most often caused by rupture of saccular aneurysms from branches of the arteries of the circle of Willis (Figure 2), but also can be caused by bleeding from arteriovenous malformations (Figure 3) and venous abnormalities. Subarachnoid hemorrhage usually presents with severe headache. "The worst headache of my life" is the common complaint. Stiff neck and photophobia also usually are present. The headache may be less severe when the aneurysm is leaking blood, rather than complete rupture. This sentinel bleed is important to recognize because it may be a warning of imminent acute rupture. Therefore, all patients presenting to an emergency department complaining of severe headache for the first time should have an emergency CT scan of the brain. If the suspicion of a subarachnoid hemorrhage is high, a lumbar puncture should be performed, even if the CT scan is negative, to rule out the presence of subarachnoid blood. A lumbar puncture is also necessary to differentiate subarachnoid hemorrhage from meningitis, which also presents with severe headache and stiff neck. When a subarachnoid hemorrhage is identified, cerebral angiography usually is performed to identify the source of bleeding. If cerebral angiography is negative, spinal cord arteriovenous malformation also should be considered.

Intraparenchymal bleeding and subarachnoid hemorrhage are neurologic catastrophes with a high morbidity and mortality rate. Immediate hospitalization is required, usually in an intensive care unit. Medical and surgical treatments are available for both conditions. Emergency surgery is preferred in subarachnoid hemorrhage.

Intraparenchymal Brain Hemorrhage

Intraparenchymal brain hemorrhage not only is primarily caused by hypertension, but also is usually accompanied by a secondary increase in blood pressure with increased intracranial pressure. The increased arterial pressure can cause continued bleeding until the intracranial pressure is equalized to cause a tamponade effect. Control of blood pressure elevation is initiated if systolic pressure is greater than 220 mm Hg or diastolic pressure is above 120 mm Hg, to attempt to contain further bleeding.[4] Reduction in blood pressure may also decrease the amount of edema that develops surrounding the hemorrhage. However, the regions of brain adjacent to the hemorrhage may become ischemic because of the pressure effect, and too great a reduction in blood pressure may decrease perfusion of viable brain tissue, resulting in irreversible ischemic damage. Intravenous labetalol (Trandate®, Normodyne®) is commonly used to titrate the blood pressure, but in severe cases of accelerated hypertension, sodium nitroprusside infusion is necessary.

Edema developing around the hemorrhage may further increase intracranial pressure. If the patient's level of consciousness is reduced, requiring endotracheal intubation, hyperventilation can be instituted to decrease the intracranial pressure. The osmotic diuretic mannitol (20% to 25% solution) can be administered intravenously with an initial dose of 1 g/kg over 30 minutes, followed by an infusion of 0.25 g/kg every 4 hours to try to prevent acute herniation.[5] Mannitol is usually only given over 24 hours, before a rebound effect with potential increased intracranial pressure occurs. Corticosteroids have not proven effective when administered to all patients with intracerebral hemorrhage.[6] Patients with large hemorrhage have a poor prognosis despite treatment, and patients with small hemorrhages do not benefit. The medical complications of corticosteroids may result in an even a worse outcome.[6] Nevertheless, intravenous dexamethasone (12 mg initially and 4 mg every 6 hours) often is administered, particularly to patients with moderate-sized intracerebral hematomas with considerable surrounding edema. The rationale for corticosteroids is that reducing the surrounding edema may in some cases preserve contiguous brain tissue and prevent herniation.

The prognosis for patients with intraparenchymal hemorrhage is related not only to the size of the hematoma, but also to the amount of intraventricular blood.[7] If the amount of intraventricular hemorrhage is large, ventriculostomy is performed to drain the blood. This also reduces the intracranial pressure, and may lessen the degree of subsequent hydrocephalus. Recent studies have demonstrated that infusion of urokinase into the ventricular system hastens the disappearance of ventricular blood.[8] A controlled trial is being instituted to determine if urokinase infusion improves outcome over ventriculostomy alone in patients with intraventricular hemorrhage.

Surgical evacuation of intracerebral hemorrhages has not been documented to be effective.[9] Although acute mortality rate may be somewhat reduced, the overall long-term outcome is not altered.[9] Surgery may have a role in superficial lobar hemorrhages with mass effect, in which surgery would not disrupt viable portions of the brain.

Surgical management is indicated in one instance: cerebellar hemorrhage with mass effect on the brain stem. Cerebellar hemorrhage can initially present as an apparently innocuous episode of vertigo or slight imbalance, but symptoms progress, either gradually with small hemorrhages, or rapidly with larger hemorrhages. The brain stem may be compressed, causing hydrocephalus by obstructing the fourth ventricle, and reducing level of consciousness. Large hemorrhages are life-threatening without surgical evacuation, while smaller hemorrhages can be managed conservatively if no significant mass effect is present.[10] Removal of the hematoma is preferable to ventriculostomy, which can cause an adverse outcome from upward herniation of the brain stem.

Subarachnoid Hemorrhage

The main arteries of the brain are situated in the subarachnoid space and do not communicate directly with the brain parenchyma. When an intracranial aneurysm ruptures, the blood often remains in the subarachnoid space, but can also dissect into the brain, causing intraparenchymal hematomas. The severity of the symptoms

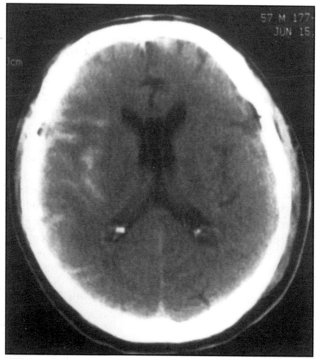

Figure 4: *Computed axial tomography of the brain demonstrates subarachnoid blood filling the sulci, which appear white from blood, rather than black as when filled with cerebrospinal fluid. Courtesy of Dr. Adam Silvers.*

is proportional to the amount of bleeding and whether focal deficits are present from intraparenchymal extension of the blood. Prognosis can be estimated from the amount of blood seen on CT scan of the brain[11] (Figure 4).

The status of the patient is most commonly graded with the Hunt-Hess Scale (Table 1).[12] Grade I represents patients with mild headache, the sentinel bleed. Grade II patients have moderate to severe headache and nuchal rigidity, but do not have any focal neurologic deficits ex-

Table 1: Hunt and Hess Clinical Grades of Subarachnoid Hemorrhage

Grade	Clinical Status
I	No symptoms, minimal headache or stiff neck
II	Severe headache, stiff neck
III	Confusion or drowsiness, mild hemiparesis
IV	Deep stupor, moderate to severe hemiparesis, early decerebrate signs
V	Coma

cept, in some cases, an oculomotor palsy. Blood in the subarachnoid space can put pressure on the oculomotor nerve, which lies just below the posterior communicating artery, a common location of aneurysms. This results in ptosis of the eyelid, dilated pupil, and paresis of upward, downward, and medial movements of the affected eye. It does not necessarily signify intraparenchymal extension of blood. However, when level of consciousness is reduced, a dilated pupil may be a sign of brain herniation. Grade III patients experience confusion, drowsiness, or mild focal signs such as a drift of the contralateral arm. Grade IV patients have a frank hemiparesis, or are stuporous and difficult to arouse. Grade V patients are comatose, unarousable, and may have signs of brain herniation with decorticate or decerebrate posturing: forced rigid extension of the legs, and either forced rigid flexion or extension of the upper extremities.

The outcome for patients with grade IV or V lesions is dismal, and no effective treatment has been developed,[13,14] but patients in grades I through III on initial presentation are still in danger. Two factors can precipitate adverse outcome in patients with mild to moderate subarachnoid hemorrhage: recurrence of bleeding and vasospasm. Bleeding can reoccur at any time after the initial event. Vasospasm begins several days after the bleed, with maximal spasm between 4 and 7 days after the initial event.[15]

Once diagnosis has been established, subarachnoid hemorrhage is initially managed by medically stabilizing the patient, and then angiography to identify the source of the bleeding. Blood pressure should be reduced to the low normal range to try to prevent rebleeding. In the early stages, ischemia from vasospasm is not a problem; however, during the phase of vasospasm, low blood pressure may result in more ischemic events. The calcium channel blocker nimodipine (Nimotop®) lowers blood pressure, reduces the ischemic consequences of vasospasm,[16] and improves overall outcome.[17] Nimodipine administered 60 mg orally (or by nasogastric tube in a patient unable to swallow) every 4 hours for 21 days reduced the incidence of ischemic stroke from spasm by 34% and poor outcome by 40%, with no increased incidence of rebleeding.[16]

Another medical strategy for prevention of rebleeding is to prevent the fibrinolysins in the cerebrospinal fluid from dissolving the clot formed at the site of the aneurysmal rupture. The antifibrinolysins aminocaproic acid (Amicar®) and tranexamic acid have been used.[18] Aminocaproic acid, 24 to 36 g/d by constant IV infusion, reduced the 7-day mortality rate from 22.6% to 12.1%, primarily by reducing rebleeding.[18] Tranexamic acid reduced the 7-day mortality rate to 8.1%. However, these agents were associated with long-term complications—an increase in cerebral ischemic events and venous thromboembolic events—and are generally not used since the advent of nimodipine therapy.

Corticosteroids have not proven effective in patients with subarachnoid hemorrhage, but are often given for signs of increased intracranial pressure. A recent trial of a steroid derivative, the 21-aminosteroid antioxidant tirilazad mesylate given intravenously 2 mg/kg, showed a positive trend for improved outcome compared with placebo in a phase II trial.[19] Anticonvulsants are usually administered because the incidence of seizures accompanying subarachnoid hemorrhage is 10%.[20]

The most definitive method for prevention of rebleeding is surgical clipping of the aneurysm. Aneurysm surgery within the 4-to-10-day period of spasm has an unacceptably high rate of complications, and should be avoided.[21] Early surgery, within the first 3 days after rupture, reduces the mortality rate, while delaying surgery between 10 and 14 days produces better surgical results and fewer postoperative neurologic deficits.[14] The overall number of good outcomes with patients recovering to relatively normal functional status was the same for both early and late surgical intervention, about 58%.[14]

The optimal treatment for patients in grades I or II appears to be immediate surgery within the first 24 hours, to prevent rebleeding without causing brain injury related to spasm during the surgery.[22] Once the aneurysm is clipped, ischemic consequences of spasm can be prevented with nimodipine.[22] Perfusion can be maintained in areas of vasospasm by plasma volume expansion using Plasmanate or hetastarch to elevate the central venous filling pressure to approximately 10 mm Hg or the pulmonary wedge pressure to 14 to 18 mm Hg.[23] If this is unsuccessful in restoring perfusion, hypertension is induced with dopamine or dobutamine to elevate the mean arterial blood pressure by 20 to 40 mm Hg.[23] The degree of vasospasm is initially assessed by angiography if the patient deteriorates clinically after clipping of the aneurysm, but can then be monitored by transcranial Doppler, which identifies increased flow velocities when spasm is present.[24] In severe cases of vasospasm, balloon angioplasty and intraarterial pharmacologic vasodilation with papaverine have been used.[25] Rebleeding will not occur with these measures once the aneurysm is clipped, but when spasm occurs in a patient waiting for surgery, perfusion cannot be increased, and nimodipine must be used.

Surgical management of aneurysms after subarachnoid hemorrhage requires manipulation of the damaged brain, which can lead to irreversible neurologic consequences. Several strategies have been developed to avoid these surgical complications. Endoscopic clipping of cerebral aneurysms can be performed to avoid traction on brain structures during the operation by performing surgery through a burr hole.[26] However, the clinician has less control of the operative field if the aneurysm ruptures during surgery.[26]

Endovascular occlusion of aneurysms with detachable platinum coils has been developed.[27] Coiling of the aneurysm is recommended in medically unstable patients or patients in poor neurologic condition, in patients with severe atherosclerosis of the parent arteries, and in recurrent aneurysms after unsuccessful surgery.[28] The drawbacks for coiling are that the recurrence rate of aneurysm formation is higher than for surgical clipping, and that the coils cannot be placed within the aneurysmal sac if the mouth of the aneurysm is wide or the feeding vessels are tortuous.[28] Coiling of aneurysms is not without complications. The rate of cerebral embolization is 3.5%, and the rate of parent artery occlusion, which can cause ischemic stroke, is 3.2%.[29] Aneurysm perforation occurs in 1.78%, causing rebleeding.[29] The overall morbidity for anterior circulation aneurysms is 9.8%, and the mortality rate is 1.8%.[29] For posterior circulation lesions, which are less accessible to surgical intervention, the morbidity was 9.6% and the mortality was 3.2%.[29] However, as with surgical treatment, most of the complications were in patients with grade IV and V clinical status.[29]

Despite the advanced surgical and interventional techniques to treat aneurysmal subarachnoid hemorrhage, the overall outcome still has an undesirably high rate of morbidity and mortality. Some researchers have maintained that nonsurgical treatment of aneurysm patients, with hypotension to the point of orthostatic postural changes, is just as effective as surgical management,[30] and this has been confirmed in the acute phase in at least one multicenter trial.[31]

Identification of unruptured aneurysms by screening patients with a family history of subarachnoid hemorrhage or with other risk factors, such as polycystic kidney, may help prevent aneurysmal subarachnoid hemorrhage.[32] Magnetic resonance angiography is a noninvasive method for aneurysm screening with acceptable accuracy for aneurysms in the circle of Willis, although more peripheral aneurysms may not be identified.[32] Incidental aneurysms may be detected on magnetic resonance imaging (MRI) or CT scanning of the brain for other indications.

The incidence of unruptured aneurysms in nonselected autopsy studies has been between 0.2% and 9.9%.[33] The risk of rupture of an asymptomatic aneurysm is about 2% a year. Larger aneurysms are more likely to rupture.[33] Aneurysms less than 6 mm may be safe to follow without surgery, but patients with aneurysms greater than 6 mm should be considered for surgical intervention.[33] However, two recent studies have suggested that the risk of surgery in asymptomatic patients may be greater than the risk of hemorrhage.[34,35]

Arteriovenous and Venous Malformations

The morbidity and mortality from arteriovenous malformations (AVMs) is lower than from cerebral aneurysms. Patients may present with symptoms of an expanding mass lesion or with seizures, rather than with symptoms of subarachnoid hemorrhage, particularly with larger AVMs.[36] The bleeding usually is venous rather than arterial, and is not as catastrophic as bleeding from aneurysms. The acute mortality rate is about 10%, and is 23%

in long-term follow-up of patients with an initial bleed,[36] compared with an approximate 50% acute mortality rate for ruptured cerebral aneurysms.

Surgical management of AVMs is difficult because complete removal often cannot be achieved, and considerable involvement of brain parenchyma can occur at surgery, resulting in neurologic deficits. Coiling of AVMs has been effective in eliminating the lesion or reducing its size so surgical removal is feasible.[37]

Stereotactic radiosurgery also has been used to fibrose the AVM,[38] with complete disappearance of the AVM at 1 year in 40% to 50% of cases, and at 2 years in 80% of cases.[38] However, neurologic complications from radiation necrosis of the brain can occur in 4% to 17% of cases.[38] Large AVMs may not be effectively treated with radiation, but a combination of coiling to reduce the size of the AVM, followed by radiosurgery, may be optimal for these patients.[38]

Cavernous malformations are abnormal collections of venous tissue filled with blood that do not communicate directly with the arterial system, as in AVMs. They generally present with intracranial hematomas, seizures, or focal neurologic deficits, but rarely present with subarachnoid hemorrhage, and often remain asymptomatic.[36] Nevertheless, about 15% of patients who present with symptoms of hemorrhage from cavernous malformations may have a poor clinical outcome.[36] Venous angiomas are sometimes identified as incidental findings on MRI or in patients with vascular headaches. They are histologically normal dilated or varicose veins that almost never produce subarachnoid hemorrhage.[36] However, they can co-exist with cavernous malformations and, when a patient with a venous angioma develops a cerebral hemorrhage, high-resolution MRI often documents the presence of a cavernous malformation.[36] Surgical management of cavernous malformations usually is not possible because they are part of the brain parenchyma.

Conclusion

Intracerebral and subarachnoid hemorrhage are catastrophic neurologic diseases that still have devastating results, despite recent technologic advances. Control of hypertension appears to be the most effective method for prevention of intracerebral hemorrhage, and may be effective in reducing the rate of aneurysmal subarachnoid hemorrhage as well. Rapid identification of patients with the warning sentinel bleed from a cerebral aneurysm affords the best opportunity for treatment before a severe subarachnoid hemorrhage occurs. Screening of high-risk individuals for aneurysms with magnetic resonance angiography also may be helpful in reducing the consequences of this dire illness.

References

1. Sherman DG, Dyken ML Jr, Gent M, et al: Antithrombotic therapy for cerebrovascular disorders. An update. *Chest* 1995; 108:444S-456S.

2. Cole FM, Yates PO: The occurrence and significance of intracerebral micro-aneurysms. *J Pathol Bacteriol* 1967;93:393-411.

3. Vinters HV: Cerebral amyloid angiopathy. A critical review. *Stroke* 1987;18:311-324.

4. National Stroke Association Consensus Statement: Stroke: the first six hours: emergency evaluation and treatment. *J Stroke Cerebrovasc Dis* 1993;3:133-144.

5. Marshall LF, Smith RW, Rauscher LA, et al: Mannitol dose requirements in brain-injured patients. *J Neurosurg* 1978;48: 169-172.

6. Poungvarin N, Bhoopat W, Viriyavejakul A, et al: Effects of dexamethasone in primary supratentorial intracerebral hemorrhage. *N Engl J Med* 1987;316:1229-1233.

7. Tuhrim S, Horowitz DR, Sacher M, et al: Validation and comparison of models predicting survival following intracerebral hemorrhage. *Crit Care Med* 1995;23:950-954.

8. Rainov NG, Burkert WL: Urokinase infusion for severe intraventricular haemorrhage. *Acta Neurochir (Wien)* 1995; 134:55-59.

9.   Hankey GJ, Hon C: Surgery for primary intracerebral hemorrhage: is it safe and effective? A systematic review of case series and randomized trials. *Stroke* 1997;28:2126-2132.

10.   Auer LM, Auer T, Sayama I: Indications for surgical treatment of cerebellar haemorrhage and infarction. *Acta Neurochir (Wien)* 1986;79:74-79.

11.   Adams HP Jr, Kassell NF, Torner JC: Usefulness of computed tomography in predicting outcome after aneurysmal subarachnoid hemorrhage: a preliminary report of the Cooperative Aneurysm Study. *Neurology* 1985;35:1263-1267.

12.   Hunt WE, Hess RM: Surgical risk as related to time of intervention in the repair of intracranial aneurysms. *J Neurosurg* 1968;28:14-20.

13.   Kassell NF, Torner JC, Haley EC Jr, et al: The International Cooperative Study on the Timing of Aneurysm Surgery. Part 1: Overall management results. *J Neurosurg* 1990;73:18-36.

14.   Kassell NF, Torner JC, Jane JA, et al: The International Cooperative Study on the Timing of Aneurysm Surgery. Part 2: Surgical results. *J Neurosurg* 1990;73:37-47.

15.   Heros RC, Zervas NT, Varsos V: Cerebral vasospasm after subarachnoid hemorrhage: an update. *Ann Neurol* 1983;14:599-608.

16.   Allen GS, Ahn HS, Preziosi TJ, et al: Cerebral arterial spasm—a controlled trial of nimodipine in patients with subarachnoid hemorrhage. *N Engl J Med* 1983;308:619-624.

17.   Pickard JD, Murray GD, Illingworth R, et al: Effect of oral nimodipine on cerebral infarction and outcome after subarachnoid haemorrhage: British aneurysm nimodipine trial. *BMJ* 1989; 298:636-642.

18.   Kassell NF, Torner JC, Adams HP Jr: Antifibrinolytic therapy in the acute period following aneurysmal subarachnoid hemorrhage. Preliminary observations from the Cooperative Aneurysm Study. *J Neurosurg* 1984;61:225-230.

19.   Haley EC Jr, Kassell NF, Alves WM, et al: Phase II trial of tirilazad in aneurysmal subarachnoid hemorrhage. A report of the Cooperative Aneurysm Study. *J Neurosurg* 1995;82:786-790.

20.   Hart RG, Byer JA, Slaughter JR, et al: Occurrence and implications of seizures in subarachnoid hemorrhage due to ruptured intracranial aneurysms. *Neurosurgery* 1981;8:417-421.

21. Graf CJ, Nibbelink DW: Cooperative study of intracranial aneurysms and subarachnoid hemorrhage. Report on a randomized treatment study. 3. Intracranial surgery. *Stroke* 1974;5:557-601.

22. Auer LM, Brandt L, Ebeling U, et al: Nimodipine and early aneurysm operation in good condition SAH patients. *Acta Neurochir (Wien)* 1986;82:7-13.

23. Kassell NF, Peerless SJ, Durward QJ: Treatment of ischemic deficits from vasospasm with intravascular volume expansion and induced arterial hypertension. *Neurosurgery* 1982;11:337-343.

24. Aaslid R, Huber P, Nornes H: Evaluation of cerebrovascular spasm with transcranial Doppler ultrasound. *J Neurosurg* 1984;60:37-41.

25. Duckwiler G: Balloon angioplasty and intra-arterial papaverine for vasospasm. *J Stroke Cerebrovasc Dis* 1997;6:261-263.

26. Frazee JG, King WA, De Salles AA, et al: Endoscopic-assisted clipping of cerebral aneurysms. *J Stroke Cerebrovasc Dis* 1997;6:240-241.

27. Guglielmi G: Endovascular treatment of aneurysms. History, development, and application of current techniques. *J Stroke Cerebrovasc Dis* 1997;6:246-248.

28. Martin NA: Decision-making for intracranial aneurysm treatment: when to select surgery, and when to select endovascular therapy. *J Stroke Cerebrovasc Dis* 1997;6:253-257.

29. Vinuela F, Duckwiler G, Guglielmi G: Guglielmi detachable coil embolization of intracranial aneurysms. *J Stroke Cerebrovasc Dis* 1997;6:249-252.

30. Slosberg PS: Unexpected results in long-term medically treated ruptured intracranial aneurysm including data on 14 patients followed more than 30 years each. *Acta Neurochir (Wien)* 1997;139:697-705.

31. Nibbelink DW: Antihypertensive and antifibrinolytic therapy following subarachnoid hemorrhage from ruptured intracranial aneurysms. In: Sahs AL, Nibbelink DW, Torner JC, eds. *Aneurysmal Subarachnoid Hemorrhage: Report of the Cooperative Study*, vol. 13. Baltimore, Urban & Schwarzenberg, 1981, pp 297-306.

32. Frazee JG, Kelly DF: Treatment of unruptured aneurysms. *J Stroke Cerebrovasc Dis* 1997;6:227-229.

33. Wiebers DO, Torner JC, Meissner I: Impact of unruptured intracranial aneurysms on public health in the United States. *Stroke* 1992;23:1416-1419.

34. Johnston SC, Dudley RA, Gress DR, et al: Surgical and endovascular treatment of unruptured cerebral aneurysms at university hospitals. *Neurology* 1999;10;52(9):1799-1805.

35. The Magnetic Resonance Angiography in Relatives of Patients with Subarachnoid Hemorrhage Study Group: Risks and benefits of screening for intracranial aneurysms in first-degree relatives of patients with sporadic subarachnoid hemorrhage. *N Engl J Med* 1999;341:1344-1350.

36. Barrow DL: Classification and natural history of cerebral vascular malformations: arteriovenous, cavernous, and venous. *J Stroke Cerebrovasc Dis* 1997;6:264-267.

37. Vinuela F, Duckwiler G, Guglielmi G: Contribution of interventional neuroradiology in the therapeutic management of brain arteriovenous malformations. *J Stroke Cerebrovasc Dis* 1997;6:268-271.

38. Martin NA: Treatment of arteriovenous malformations: indications, grading, and techniques. *J Stroke Cerebrovasc Dis* 1997;6:272-276.

Index

B

C